THE GIFT
OF
LYME DISEASE
AND
CO-INFECTIONS

A Healer's Journey
to Healing Lyme

Suzen Chan

Got Lyme? Get Answers

www.TheGiftOfLymeDisease.com
and
www.SuzenChanHealthCounselor.com

BALBOA
PRESS
A DIVISION OF HAY HOUSE

Balboa Press books may be ordered through booksellers or by contacting:

Balboa Press
A Division of Hay House
1663 Liberty Drive
Bloomington, IN 47403
www.balboapress.com
1 (877) 407-4847

Print information available on the last page.

ISBN: 978-1-5043-6696-0 (sc)
ISBN: 978-1-5043-6697-7 (hc)
ISBN: 978-1-5043-6722-6 (e)

Library of Congress Control Number: 2016916013

Balboa Press rev. date: 10/17/2016

For

my divine shining stars

I will instruct you and teach you
In the way you should go; I will
Counsel you and watch over you.

—Psalm 32:8

ACKNOWLEDGMENTS

THANK YOU TO all my friends and family who watched over me during this very dark and difficult part of my life. You were kind, patient, compassionate and loving when I needed you most. Thank you from the very bottom of my Heart.

Thank you to all the doctors and medical staffers and healers who did their best to help me find a cure. Your ability to hold the focus of wellness for me when I could not, was monumental. I will always have a place of gratitude in my Heart for you.

Thank you to all my Angels and Messengers sent from Heaven to guide me along this healing path. You are all loved and appreciated.

Thank you to Sophia and Jesus, my Lord God and Savior. The healing works contained in the Bible were essential to unlocking the secret laws of health.

MISSION STATEMENT

To move through this world with congruent integrity
as a compassionate influencing catalyst for self-
empowerment with a focus on reclaiming authentic
health and vitality through love joy and gratitude.

The cure of many diseases
Is unknown to physicians …
Because they are ignorant of the whole.
For the part can never be well
Unless the whole is well.

—Plato

TABLE OF CONTENTS

PREFACE

LYME DISEASE IS an insufferable disease. Recent reports claim 300,000 people a year are struck down by Lyme disease and co-infections.

This rising epidemic involves astronomical costs in terms of lost:

employment
schooling
health
wealth
joy
happiness
tranquility
relationships
physical activity
ability to thrive
standard of living
loss of driving ability and independence
long-term joy for life
goals
memory loss
hearing
smelling
visual acuity
taste
confidence in life
articulate speech control
loss of confidence with medical system
social events
social graces
friends

personal growth stagnates
While increasing these unwanted attributes:
weight gain or weight loss
depression
sleep disturbance
emotional rages
damage to heart
damage to nervous system
rashes
imbalance vertigo
medication side effects
hallucinations
compounding chronic pain
endless searching for answers with no solution
death in some instances

And it drags on for years. For the individual affected, it is an acute and sub-acute roller-coaster ride requiring long distance endurance. Ultimately acceptance and surrender allow us to find a thorough and permanent solution with Mother Nature as our guide.

With so many falling ill and lost within the confusion of insurance company policies and failing medical protocols, the future seems bleak.

I am here to say there is a way!

I did it and you can too.

There *are* answers.

Recovery *is* possible.

The answers are *simple* but they are not always *easy*.

It is my intent to share my personal experience of recovery from Lyme disease against all odds after the official doctors report stated I would never work again. It was a long road with many lessons. I hope there is something here within these pages that will aid you in your own recovery or that of a loved one.

This opportunity to see deep within an illness is profoundly eye-opening. What I found most intriguing was the cross-association of so many topics that are seemingly disconnected. The chronically ill patient comes to the realization we live in a toxic world today. Everything is interwoven. You cannot discuss optimum health without addressing food and lifestyle choices. You cannot explore Lyme disease without discussing the draining issues of politics, economics and environmental turmoil, all presenting blocks on the way to healing.

Organized and refined individual health regimes further our own ability to selfheal. Now, going forward, certain choices may require a change in how we make decisions based on the results of these choices.

As part of the Lyme community, heavily weighing in on the policies and governmental programs that affect us most can come at a great cost too early on in personal and individual recovery processes. During my years of recovery I witnessed passionate people who were suffering greatly from Lyme. Instead of investing their focus and energy on self healing, they rather spent their precious energy on arguing about conspiracy plots and pointing fingers at who they believed was to blame for their plight. Today these same people are stuck in the round file of chronic Lyme disability.

The fact is there is much one needs to do on the self care front to move healing along. If the medical community just discovered last year that the brain has a lymphatic system, do you really want to take a passive approach to your own healing journey?

Prioritization of outstanding health and wellness efforts early on is necessary in order to create a deeper and more positive impact in our personal world of recovery. Once we have regained our health status, we will then have the experience and stamina to weigh in on the political side. To do both at the same time will delay ones healing.

INTRODUCTION

"LET'S SEE IF you get sick." Incredulously, I turned to look at the dismissive medical attendant who, unbeknownst to me, had just sealed my fate, marrying me to the greatest physical health challenge I have ever endured.

The journey of chronic neurological Lyme disease, which very nearly killed me, was totally preventable. Instead, it devoured my precious life source for years.

Sadly and disturbingly, I was to discover the horrifying truth that I was not alone in the dismal mess of chronic Lyme disease and co-infections.

Every year over 300,000 people are diagnosed with Lyme disease. Countless others suffer misdiagnosis, ridicule, and misunderstanding. They struggle to find a cure for the pain and suffering.

Many of us carry long-held patterns and emotional blocks that prevent the purest expression of our souls receptivity for healing. Taking the time to work through these issues as they arise in the healing journey is essential.

Throughout my years of recovery I learned to embrace levity as a spirit to cultivate. I learned to laugh at myself, and with those around me, at far out ideas such as tin foil hats and aluminum meditation balls, and oh the peels of laughter when the topic of enemas arises! There are often times when we try something only to find out later it was not what we needed at all. Instead of getting depressed I would give myself a hug for best effort and go on to try the next tool.

Eventually, it was through my own empirically based trial-and-error results of incorporating each next solution presented in front of me that

I found my way back to health and along the way the Gift of Lyme disease.

Somehow it all comes out right in the end as we begin to appreciate our very own unique imprint and the clues that reveal who we are and how we fit intricately and intimately into this world of Mother Nature.

It is amazing and exciting when we start to address our needs with Mother Nature's traditional common-sense remedies and we experience positive results. With so many options to choose from, we are required to be our own best advocate when taking the full ride back to health and vitality.

One key is to reframe negative thoughts and thus eliminate resistance in order to achieve alignment with perfect health. Empathize and reframe with the Spirit of Love when others are discouraging and destroying hope.

CHRONIC LYME IS REAL

AFTER YEARS OF struggling with pain, despair and the frustration of trying to find the way back to full health, the dark cloud of depression drives many in our community to consider suicide.

Throughout the years of the Lyme healing journey, it served me well to strive for self-empowerment. Now when I work with people recovering from Lyme, I encourage them to be willing to take charge, step up in leadership and to add to the light of the world. Having Lyme, one is tested with a continual stream of insults and assaults upon the heart, soul, mind and body.

Eventually chronic Lyme forces one to examine and stop all draining behaviors like people pleasing, which do not serve ones immediate recovery.

These behaviors wear one down and deplete precious energy necessary for recovery. Eventually we learn it makes more sense to heal ourselves first, before ever giving our finite and precious life-source energy over to another.

Sensitive, multi-tasking, highly functioning, high-performing people are struck down by Lyme disease and co-infections, often leaving them without an end-game strategy.

Lost in the world of medicine, Lyme sufferers look for a way out of the pain. It is a mousetrap of nonsensical paths leading to frustration at every turn.

It is an enemy invisible to the naked eye. Casual onlookers cannot comprehend the abject terror-filled pain which continually wracks our body, mind, and spirit. Self-doubt creeps in as we, too, wonder if it is really all in our head. As the years drag on and the illness drives in deeper, desperation grows.

Soft-tissue inflammation causes further damage as the bacteria build their colonies by incorporating heavy metal deposits within our body resulting in bio-film complexes. For some, when this strikes as with a gut-wrenching assault on the digestive track, we are alone in this crippling grip.

Others endure thunder-and-lightning, mind-exploding headaches which can be followed directly by an abrupt disconnect and shutoff of access to our memory and/or ability to articulate.

Speech becomes impaired, with words floating just out of reach, yet within sight, as we struggle to express coherent thoughts.

The brain-to-mouth cue has blown a circuit. We are left standing frozen like a deer in the headlights.

Driving down familiar roads can become a terrifying experience of amnesia.

One looses control of ones own body over time. It becomes a carcass existing in servitude to the whims and demands of the demon plague called Lyme disease and co-infections.

I currently assist people in finding their gift in their struggle through recovery. Why would someone want to find a gift? What will it lead to? How do we know it is a gift? Who should take this journey?

I cured myself of Lyme. There is a gift in the end.

Make no mistake it left a lot of damage in its wake.

It took five years of intensive effort and research to reverse the negative prognosis the doctors claimed was to be my future.

I started keeping a journal to communicate with this illness early on. I started seeing this sickness as a need to reclaim a more positive approach to healing. Instead of seeing this sickness as an enemy that must be annihilated, I designated the illness as my opponent in a game of strategy similar to chess.

Energy cannot be destroyed; it can only be miraculously transformed. That miracle emerges from our own thoughts. It is our own personal decision when to release ourselves from being entrapped by lonely fear and anger built on past wounds.

We should rather embrace a view of the world that is grounded in hope, love, and faith. There is certainly nothing to lose, no risk in trying.

God does his part when we do ours.

Even though I could not concentrate nor focus enough to read during my bedridden years, just knowing there were others who recovered gave me much needed hope to continue searching for relief.

It is my hope that this book will be one of those signposts for you and others to continue on with your own search for wellness.

May God bless you.

WHAT IS LYME DISEASE AND CO-INFECTIONS?

LYME DISEASE IS caused by a bite from a black legged deer tick that has been infected with the bacteria *Borrelia burgdorferi*. Both humans and animals can be infected with this disease, but not all ticks carry this disease and not everyone who gets a tick bite contracts Lyme disease.

Symptoms may vary from headaches, arthritis, joint pain, extreme fatigue, muscle aches and pains, flu-like symptoms, vomiting, all the way to meningitis neck pain and fever. Some people who have been bitten by a Lyme tick develop a bullseye rash, others do not, or they develop them years later. If you experience a tick bite or bullseye rash please go immediately to have your doctor confirm through testing if you have contracted Lyme disease or any co-infections. The sooner you start treating Lyme and co-infections the better and speedier your recovery will be.

Here is the bad thing though, of the approximately 33 different types of Lyme bacteria, testing for only two or three different types of bacteria is presently available. It is also known ticks can carry co-infections such as Bartonella, borreliosis, anaplasmosis, babesiosis, and *B. miyamotoi* infection.

And the other bad news — these test results are often not accurate.

There is talk that Lyme disease may be a combination of virus and bacteria. Lyme was originally classified as a virus back in 1974 upon its discovery in Connecticut and then later reclassified as a bacteria. Medicine states there are no treatments for viruses but for bacteria, we have antibiotics for those who choose.

Many good reports on the TV news or in newspapers discuss tick bite prevention.

Reminding you to always tuck in:

sleeves into gloves

pant legs into socks and boots

hair covered, braided or tied in bun

shirts close fitting to the body and tucked in

boots, knee high rubber is my favorite

hats with brim

Spraying with essential oils or a natural bug defense goes a long way to keeping everyone safe.

Not everyone who is bitten contracts Lyme. Others who contract it do not remember a bite or seeing a tick. It is also congenital which means a mother can pass it on to the fetus during pregnancy. There is a suspicion it maybe sexually transmitted as well.

Ticks are everywhere, especially in moist, dark landscapes of leaves and uncut grass. Following outdoor activities, it is suggested one remove all clothing as soon as possible, shower, and inspect the entire body with the aid of a mirror or another person. Ticks like to crawl up to the base of the neck, armpits, and groin but they can attach anywhere.

Lyme disease is often misdiagnosed as ALS, Multiple Sclerosis, Parkinson, ADHD, chronic fatigue, or fibromyalgia and more. Anyone with these diagnoses should test to be sure and rule out that it is not Lyme disease. Do not be surprised if there is resistance to this testing. One may experience three stages of Lyme disease. If it can be caught early, chances of full recovery are best.

Possible early symptoms could be a bite site developing within three to thirty days, evidence of a red bulls-eye rash (erythema migraines), deep fatigue, chills, fever, headache, body aches, and swollen lymph nodes.

Additional symptoms could be rashes on other areas of the body, Bell's palsy resulting in the loss of muscle tone on one or both sides of the face, severe headaches, neck stiffness, meningitis, pain, swelling in the large joints, shooting pains, sleep disturbance, heart palpitations, vertigo, and many others.

Some of these symptoms will resolve over a period of weeks to months even without treatment. However, lack of treatment can result in additional complications.

Late-stage symptoms may emerge months to years post-tick bite and may be experienced as arthritis, muscle pains, cognitive difficulties, neurological problems, sleep disturbances, fibromyalgia, and chronic fatigue.

Q. If you do get bitten by a tick or show Lyme-like symptoms, what should you do?

A. Remove the tick properly by grabbing the tick with tweezers or a tick key at the mouth where it is attached to the skin. Most important, do not squeeze the body of the tick to avoid propelling bacteria from the ticks stomach into the host.

A Lyme-literate doctor will most likely treat you with a short course of antibiotics, optimally for thirty days. This time frame may vary slightly from case to case. You may have to press on to convince your doctor of the need for the prescription.

The earlier you receive treatment the better the chances of reversing symptoms. If you do not catch Lyme disease early, it can go years and decades undiagnosed or misdiagnosed. Most medical doctors do not believe chronic Lyme exists.

I am here to tell you that chronic neurological Lyme disease absolutely does exist.

Two tests available are the Western Blot or ELISA test. Western Blot is favored in the industry. Many providers will say testing is not necessary. Many will resist authorizing treatments as well, even with marginal evidence of Lyme.

Specific bands will show up positive on a Western Blot test for Lyme disease. Centers for Disease Control and Prevention (CDC) regulations require tests showing a certain number of positive bands to be positively diagnosed as Lyme; however, those of us who understand Lyme know that even if you only have one band show up and you have symptoms, it could be directly related to the Lyme bacteria *Borrelia burgdorferi*.

Long-term antibiotic use for Lyme has not yet been unilaterally approved. If you have chronic Lyme, you very well may have a difficult time getting the treatment you need unless you have a Lyme-literate medical doctor (LLMD) or International Lyme and Associated Diseases Society (ILADS) doctor on your team.

Locating LLMD or ILADS doctors remains challenging. Many keep a low profile to avoid being harassed by the American Medical Association mainly due to the controversy over chronic Lyme treatment with long-term antibiotics. Many doctors have had their medical licenses challenged, too many times, successfully.

Chronic Lyme treatments tend to be long, painful, distressing processes, quite often with poor outcomes. The bacteria are corkscrew-shaped spirochetes that drill into bone, cartilage, organs, and deeply into the tissues, all the places where medication cannot go.

There are many different treatment styles, starting with long-term antibiotics. With each physician choosing his or her own favored protocol, it is important to choose a doctor who will listen to you and respect what you are comfortable with concerning treatments.

Patients receiving blood transfusions should consider that it might be taking a big risk. Donated blood is not screened for Lyme or co-infections.

There is no guarantee all of the symptoms will be reversed with treatment. After a long period of time dealing with the crisis of Lyme, there is a significant amount of damage left behind. The goal is to keep improving overall wellness. It is possible to address the progression of chronic Lyme disease with proactive lifestyle choices.

All microbes exist in the presence of God and are members of the Universe. They have existed for millions of years and will continue to exist for still millions of years more to come. They are a creative force of nature. It is the toxins they produce within our body that, over time, lead to disease when they become hitchhikers in our body.

In that we are all one with the Universe it is important to maintain strong boundaries between self and other. This failure to differentiate self from other is one reason chronic illness can settle in. In this case we focus on exactly how we identify the disease, and the relationship it has to us, as an important definition. Properly pronounced "Lyme," and not "Lyme's" disease is one step towards identifying just exactly what our focus will be trained on.

These bacteria are living beings communicating with each other from their own hiding places in and around the body. As a healer I realized one cannot conduct an all-out war to aggressively kill all of these microbes without harming ones own self in the process.

I recognized there should be a strategic and systematic process to complete the task of eliminating every last Lyme bacterium. The bottom line is protocol tools need to be used in the right order, or they will not work.

Healing Lyme requires the ability to stand in faith, surrender the desire for annihilation and revenge. It commands moving through the healing process with grace.

Lyme disease can be incredibly complex and elusive. It invades organs, bones, and cartilage—basically, all the places medication cannot go. There it forms a cyst and replicates within that cyst. When these cysts burst open, what was once one spirochete, has now become seven or more. This is why Lyme can survive for years in spite of antibiotic therapy. The spirochetes remain alive but dormant in their non-accessible hiding places while the medication is in the body. Once the medication is no longer present, the spirochetes come out and play.

The problem is further complicated by political arguing and ego-puffing and dodgy insurance motives which then interferes with the medical community's ability to find an effective cure.

WHERE DO WE GO FROM HERE?

LYME DISEASE IS both demanding and damaging. Events, tasks, and everyday habits that were once taken for granted prior to getting sick become nearly impossible to attend or accomplish.

During these darker times I would refocus my efforts and meditate. I would lay or sit quietly in a darkened room, do cleansing breaths and envision my wise body healing itself. I would repeat positive statements. Here is a useful list to help you remember to walk on the sunny side of the street when there is an avalanche of stuff coming toward you.

- The goal is healing through self-empowerment.
- Conscious choices require the willingness to take full responsibility for individual lifestyle and health choice outcomes. Otherwise known as, consequences of the actions.
- Cultivation and refinement of daily lifestyle habits and nutritional choices dictate either support toward the build-up of health or facilitate the tear-down of health and life force.
- There is a gift in each struggle.
- The healing journey starts with acceptance and surrender.
- 'Blaming others takes the focus off you.' This deflecting tactic wastes precious life-force energy that is needed to replenish your own healing reserves. In other words, work to own your emotional blocks.
- The clearer and stronger you become, the more on purpose your life will be.
- The purpose of life is to discover our gifts and share them with others.
- This work is part of the journey.
- Hold the vision of vitality, health, happiness and joy.

- What are you willing to do to overcome Lyme disease and co-infections?
- Seek, ask, and pray, and it shall be.
- Where is our surrender point?
- Enhance the personal wellness journey with gratitude!

GIFT OF LYME MEDITATIONS

MOST DAYS WITH Lyme are full of pain and struggle. These are some of my favorite mantra meditations for raising energy levels to support the soul during desperate stretches of time.

- When God wants to give you a gift, he wraps it in a problem
- The bigger the problem, the bigger the gift
- Pressure makes diamonds
- The answer is within
- A grain of sand creates a pearl
- Our gift is within our struggle
- For the butterfly's wings to be strong enough to fly and soar, the emergence from its cocoon must be done alone, without intervention
- The deeper the roots grow down into the mud, the more beautiful the blossom
- God never gives us anything more than we can handle
- Believe in the power of prayer
- Ask, and you shall receive
- I am not the dis-ease of Lyme
- I am well
- I am loved
- I am whole

Keeping these reminders close at hand helps ease the struggle of maintaining balance when being ill and low:

- Take baby steps to crawl out of despair
- Develop an end-game plan for regaining a high-performance, healthy lifestyle

- Challenge yourself to remain unattached to the outcome
- Breathe in deeply, hold, exhale deeply, and repeat
- I am thankful for the things I have learned from my healing struggle: patience, perseverance, compassion and love.
- I am thankful for humor
- Laughter is better than tears
- Fake it until you make it
- Tears are the coins of healing
- I am thankful for friends who have come to witness me on this path
- I am thankful for family and friends who have aided me, even when we did not know what the problem was
- I am thankful for hope and faith and all the wonderful people

THE LESSONS OF LYME DISEASE AND HOW IT TAUGHT ME WHAT A HEALING JOURNEY IS REALLY ALL ABOUT

AS THE DAWN of wellness started to dance around me, just out of reach of Lyme misery, the beginning messages of hope first came as a whisper, most imperceptible. They sounded like this:

Do you know that with proper nutrition, detoxification, and a healthy lifestyle you can live your life in such a way as to prevent, stabilize, or eliminate chronic illness?

Do you know it starts with your surrender? Do you even know what surrender really is?

Surrender is the ability to let go again, and again, and again, and even yet again …and yes, even again.

Reach out and hold my hand, for I will lead you to the promised land. A gift is there for you to see: a loving blessing for thee.

Harmony and Whole Health Is the Gift of Life

—Suzen

Your body is your vehicle which enables you to move around and explore this beautiful garden of life we call Earth. Our bodies require regular maintenance and quality care in order to achieve quality longevity.

People often take better care of their cars then they do their physical being.

They spend more money on vacations instead of on preventative healthcare.

Reverence, respect, accountability, and compassion all play a vital role in maintaining Mother Earth's bountiful garden, which has been entrusted to us in stewardship. If Mother Earth is sick, so to, will we be sick.

My goal is to move through this world with congruent integrity and to be a compassionate catalyst motivating and influencing others toward their own self-empowerment.

In this lifetime I have overcome the diagnosis of full disability from Lyme disease and co-infections. The official doctors court report stated I would never work again. My situation was to be covered by workman's compensation which only added another layer of stress to my already taxed life. It took more than five years and every ounce of strength I had but I did thankfully overcome this disability.

In my life I have faced other great challenges as well. My choice for each situation was always to be a victor and not a victim as I moved through the aftermath of situations past.

I work with Jesus and Sophia for protection, wisdom, compassion and guidance. Prior to Lyme my paths involved studies of Alchemy in Bohemia. I became influenced by the works of Rudolf Steiner, Robert Powell, Christopher Bamford, Nicholas Goodrick-Clarke, Paracelsus, Saint Germain, and so many more.

Guidance also brought me to study with the nomads and the monks in Tibet and China, enhancing my ability to work with energetic distance healing.

All of this has been grounded with licenses in therapeutic massage and bodywork in both Connecticut and New York. Studies in Public Policy at Trinity College and, prior to that, I worked in the corporate world with IBM in Tarrytown, New York, and Princeton, New Jersey.

Once Lyme entered the picture in June 2007, everything in my life changed drastically.

Life has been challenging for me in general, but I have always managed to work through whatever has come my way. For example in 1975 our family home was devastated by a fire while we slept. This incident claimed the lives of my father and sister. It was a long time ago, but it was an event that took part of my heart along with it.

I bring this topic up for you now, not to provoke a sadness for me from you, but to broaden your understanding of what healing from Lyme involves. Especially when you are dealing with insurance companies who will stop at nothing to try and discredit their sick applicant to avoid paying out funds for treatments. You must be ready and willing to review all traumas and tragedies in your past with an ultra fine tooth comb.

When tragedies have not been addressed they leave energy cysts within the body which block energy flow. It is evident if one has done the work around such traumas. When speaking about such past events there will be an even paced openness and willingness to be vulnerable and answer all querent questions to their satisfaction.

That tragic family of origin event resulted in PTSD which later erupted and disrupted my married family life in the early '90s. PTSD can sometimes take up to twenty years to manifest symptoms, as history builds upon itself, compounding the internal pressure. Then one day something happens, you may not even perceive, say the slope of someones shoulder, a scent, anything associated with the tragedy and that will set off PTSD symptoms.

With lots of therapy and patience I was able to have a breakdown for a breakthrough in relation to this tragic event and its impact upon my life nearly 20 years after the original event, and well before Lyme hit the scene. The healer in me emerged as I healed my heart and I became a full-time licensed massage therapist.

By 2006, as I entered my fifties, life was balanced and enjoyable. Then along came Lyme in 2007 and devastated all that I had built and rebuilt in my life.

Once again I lost everything and was forced to reach deep within myself for the answers.

During my recovery from Lyme I acquired other Lyme healing skills including cranial-sacral therapy; colon hydrotherapy; flower essences, Iridology, detox and rejuvenation specialist, integrated nutrition, super-foods, herbs, and pure body and household cleansers as I learned of their benefits for healing. I never stop learning.

These skills and areas of knowledge were added to my already strong background in therapeutic massage, hypnotherapy, energy healing, yoga, pastoral counseling, gestalt/bio-energetic therapy, and aromatherapy. The combination of all these healing arts became my strength in recovery.

I still work on myself every day to be the best that I can be. Some days are better than others. I work well with people who are also interested in living a life of congruent integrity and self-responsibility.

My combined personal experience and training in gestalt/bio-energetic therapy and spiritual pastoral counseling, together helped me relate with compassion to those I work with, as we delve deep into their personal healing journey.

Holistic health coaching drives the engine of recovery, creating a solid framework for lifestyle health habits to enhance the quality of our longevity. After all, what is the point of living longer if we have a compromised state of health?

So, what is your story? What has your journey been about? Please consider. Let's make sure you know that you are *not* your issues. Rather, know you are one of God's beloved here for your fullest expression.

Certifications

- Certified Holistic Health Practitioner (CHHP)
- American Association of Drugless Practitioners (AADP)
- Certified Hypnotherapist - Hypnodyne Foundation
- Iridology - International School of Detoxification
- Detoxification and Rejuvenation Specialist - International School of Detoxification
- Cranial Sacral - Upledger Institute
- Vortex Healing - The Vortex Healing Institute
- Colon Hydrotherapy, CHT - CT Healing Institute
- Pastoral Counseling - St Francis Care of Hartford, CT
- Acupressure - CCMT
- Reflexology - American Reflexology Certification
- Therapeutic Massage - CCMT
- Immersion Fire Walker - Robbins Research Institute
- Mastery University - Robbins Research Institute
- Leadership Academy - Robbins Research Institute
- NLP - Neuro-Linguistic Programming
- Yoga Instructor Certification - Yoga-fit
- Thai-Yoga Bodywork - Vedic Conservatory
- Reiki - Usui Shiki Ryoho
- Aromatherapy Essential Oils - Scholl's School of Aromatherapy
- Flower Essences - Delta Gardens
- Diamond Palm Energetic Healing - Tibet, China, independent studies with nomads and monks
- Alchemical Studies, Czech Republic - NY Open Center, Independent Studies

- Gestalt Bio-Energetic Therapy - CT Center for Human Growth and Development
- Licensed Massage Therapist, New York and Connecticut - Connecticut Center for Massage Therapy - CCMT
- Public Policy - Trinity College

Associations

- American Association of Drugless Practitioners
- National Certification Board for Therapeutic Massage and Bodywork (NCBTMB)
- Lyme.org
- Flower Essence Society

MY STORY

JUNE 25, 2007, was the day I received my challenge from the Universe. Within a very short period of time it arrived like a high-speed freight train, literally knocking me down and out beyond all knowing, this impossible-to-penetrate foe.

This is my story of recovery from chronic neurological Lyme disease and co-infections, a healers journey of development where I clarified my comprehension as to what a healthy lifestyle *really* looks like and the meaning behind it all.

By many accounts I was already living a healthy lifestyle with clean eating, positive thinking, positive social groups, fresh air, sunshine, enjoyable employment, and regular self-examination. I was living a high-functioning lifestyle pursuing the art of healthful bliss.

I did the work—you know, the kind of dredging through the muck and mire of those dark inner canals, the 'dark night of the soul' journey.

Finally my ship seemed right-side up, and I was walking on the sunny side of the street. At fifty-one, I finally had the bounce back in my step and a smile in my eyes from knowing all the tough stuff was behind me.

Finally, life was good again!

Be aware that the Universe is always listening. I am a born seeker. From the top of the mountain to the bottom of the ocean, I have been out there seeking truth. Who and where was God? What is my purpose? Is there more I should be doing? Knock, knock. Who's there? Answer: It is your special delivery with your next assignment from Universal Source.

And there it was on that June morning in 2007, a speck the size of a grain of sand on my outer thigh as I massaged myself in my daily self care health ritual.

Hmmm, that wasn't there yesterday. I couldn't brush it off. I couldn't scratch it off. It didn't itch or hurt. I'd never seen anything like it on myself before, nor had I ever seen it on any of my massage clients in nearly twenty years as a massage therapist. After a few more swipes with no results, I continued to dress and get ready for work.

Ah, yes, work, memories. I heave a big sigh now with a bundle of mixed emotions between regret and appreciation for the "yet-to-evolve" journey I did not know lay ahead of me.

Have you ever had one of those periods in your life where you know what you want to do, but what feels right and good is exactly the opposite of what you know others, like well-meaning family, want and expect from you? Yes, that challenging fork in the road, where we must choose between wants, needs and passionate desires. Allow me to continue.

I had been happily self-employed as a massage therapist licensed in both New York and Connecticut. In this creative and demanding pursuit one must be ready to flow with each situation and outcome, come what may. In this solo profession there are no end of the year bonuses, no guarantees of any kind, for the fact is, if you do not show up, you do not get paid. Every day is different, new and challenging.

I had a professional career. I was an entrepreneur and a multiple modality healer and a good one. Most of my clients had been with me since the beginning of my practice.

In 2007, I was in a period of reviewing my professional goals and revising my long-term business plans. Because I have always had an immense curiosity about the world around me, I enjoy continually learning, traveling, and I continually challenge myself to develop new skills and talents. Therefore, my healing abilities had evolved and by now I had grown beyond massage therapy. I was more than simply a massage therapist.

Along the way I also developed an appreciation for the importance of marketing, administrative skills and networking skills required to run a fully rounded business. Presently, my curiosity and yearning for growth had me wanting to expand my role. I hadn't worked in a corporate office environment for decades. With that in mind, plus family pressure, I decided it would be a good idea to apply for a staff position at an upstate holistic summer camp for adults. My duties as program coordinator were divided between administrative computer desk work and walking all across campus to ensure rooms were set as per speakers and teachers requirements. It was an exciting job at a meaningful facility with mindful people. Woo-hoo! What could possibly go wrong?

Was this flawed thinking on my part? Hard to say. In retrospect it may seem so, because as a direct result of having this job, I contracted Lyme disease, which then infiltrated and ruined my life.

In my desire to re-enter the business world with a reference, I volunteered in exchange for learning updated office skills. Who knew what this exciting new world would bring and what new adventures I would experience!

Of all the places I have traveled around the world at great personal risk, nothing bad has ever happened to me in any of those places.

Take for instance the multiple times I have traveled to China and Tibet. The journeys to Tibet took me to places at elevations of fourteen thousand feet. We traveled on horseback, ate, slept, lived, and studied with the nomads and studied with the monks in the deeply mountainous regions of Tibet accessed only by horseback. There I learned Buddhism by the seat of my pants, so to speak.

There were no hospitals, helicopters, cities, or towns. There were only small encampments sporadically sprinkled here and there; perhaps we would see one every few days as we traveled from monastery to monastery.

Before I committed to these travels I had to accept the fact that if anything were to happen to me, we were as far away from help as one could get, and I could possibly die. I traveled with a team of ten men for these recording expeditions. I reasoned that I was traveling with healers and those of deep faith. I believed that if anything happened to me, they would have the skills and knowledge to tend to anything I might need. In all my years of worldly travel to other destinations, this has always been true as well. I have never had a problem.

Now I had to wonder at this disease taking my entire life down to the ground level on my own home turf. What happened? How could this happen in the United States with the best medicine in the world?

Up to this point I had barely heard about Lyme disease. I remember seeing a documentary in the 1980s covering fetal damage due to an active Lyme infection in the mother while pregnant. I did not appreciate the depth of this disability nor the pain and destruction such disease carries with it. I assumed one would just get over it with medication.

My perception from watching the 1980s documentary was that fetal damage occurred because Lyme disease was undetected and untreated. The conclusion was that once detected and treated it would present no further problem. When I was bitten by a deer tick in June 2007, however, I found out just how vigilant one needs to be in order to recover and protect ones precious state of health.

Thankfully, I was focused on these truths way before this almost unbeatable illness knocked at my door. As a high-functioning multiple modality bodyworker and healing therapist, I was already using tools and techniques to maintain my holistic wellness through nutrition and lifestyle. Eventually I was to draw on these roots in a much more comprehensive and deeper way in order to achieve my full recovery.

The reality, however, was that no matter how healthy I was, I wasn't healthy enough to defend against this wily, dastardly, and potent foe.

LESSON #1: DON'T GIVE YOUR POWER AWAY

I FOUND THE tick bite while massaging myself during my daily health maintenance routine. When I discovered the tiny marked bump, it was like a grain of sand in my outer right thigh. Realizing it had not been there the day before, I feared it was a tick bite but since I had never been bitten before I was unsure.

This was where the "nightmare meets Keystone cops" part of my Lyme journey began.

During our volunteer orientation meeting for my new job, we were warned that there was a lot of Lyme on the campus. We were told to look out for bites on our body; if we found one, we were to immediately go to the medical office and have one of the medical attendants remove it because the removal needed to be done in a particular way.

Immediately after discovering the suspected bite on my leg, I went into the medical office to confirm and identify this possible tick bite.

Shockingly, I was treated dismissively by the medical staff. The attendant on duty casually looked at the bite on my leg from across the room while reclining in his desk chair.

From more than six feet away he claimed, "No, that's not a tick bite."

I said, "Really? Because you're looking sideways—from across the room—and I'm looking down at it, and it looks like it's burrowed in."

To that, the attendant replied, "Nope, ticks don't burrow in". I was very confused and I'm not one to make waves so I accepted his 'professional' diagnosis and headed for the door. As I put my hand on the door knob to leave, his parting words were "… let's see if you get sick."

I did a double take as I was leaving the office at this incredible parting comment. But by then the attendant had turned his attention back to something on the desk, and I had been dismissed.

As I stepped out into the reception room, I spotted the nurse in attendance behind the reception counter casually chatting with a visitor. I summoned her attention and asked her "Do you think this is a tick?" as I lifted my garment and exposed the bite on my outer thigh. She viewed it from across the counter and, like the medical attendant, without performing a close-up examination, was very dismissive and nonchalant. She also claimed it was not a tick.

Now many of you can be heard saying, " *Of course ticks burrow in!*"

Well, I didn't know for sure. I *thought* so, but I'd never been bitten before, and I'd only seen ticks in photos.

Fast forward a week and a half. Yes, I did end up getting sick. The symptoms came over me like a freight train slamming full force into a brick wall. By Friday morning I was not feeling so good … and, wow, did I get sick fast.

MY SYMPTOMS

I HAD BEEN feeling well enough for the week and half following the suspected bite and prompt dismissal from the medical staff. During that following week a tiny black speck appeared at this grain of sand bump site and fell off by itself soon after I found it.

My healthy lifestyle changed in an instant. Once the symptoms developed within the following week they never let up. Lyme was too much for my body to withstand.

Just about a week and a half from the date of the bite, I began to develop a fever, which is unusual for me. I also experienced vertigo, occipital (cervical neck) pain, and sacral (tailbone) pain.

There was also a strange accompanying vibrating humming sensation of being outside my body, like watching myself from beside myself. At one point I commented to a co-worker that it felt like I was in a bad government experiment. I was as shocked at my own comment, as was my co-worker, who exclaimed, "Wow, it's that bad?"

Now, nearly two weeks later, with my newly developing fever and symptoms, I returned to the same medical office for help. This time there was a new medical attendant on this day. Keeping count, we are up to three medical people "helping" me during these vital and early critical stages of Lyme disease.

She took my temperature, which was 101.3, declared I had the cold that was going around campus, and asked if I would like some cold medication.

I told her I did not think it was a cold, given the accompanying spinal pains, and I said that I had also recently been bitten by a tick. I told her the bite had been dismissed earlier by the two medical staff and had not been examined or removed. She *also refused to look at the bite*. She insisted it was a cold and sent me back to my desk.

By now my symptoms were advancing rapidly, as I negotiated the hallway back to my desk. I felt a wave of nausea pass over me as the delirium from the increasing fever rendered me grossly unstable. It was a strange and dreamlike state.

In a panic, as the wave of nausea began to pick up momentum, I grabbed the nearest bucket and stumbled into the main supply closet. Just as I was about to deliver the goods, a coworker opened the door and walked into me. It was one of those movie moments where the two characters scream "AAHHH" at each other as they try to recover from startling one another.

This ruckus brought the boss from his office. "What's going on here?" I told him about my situation and that I was feeling sick. "Well, then, go back to your cabin and lie down," he said in a huff before turning and leaving.

I barely made the solo mini-commute across the campus back to the sanctity of my cabin bed.

That was Friday morning. By Sunday the nurse and staff finally came looking for me. I had been lying in bed for three days alone and unchecked, in and out of consciousness, mostly out of conscious, with a raging meningitis fever, very severe neck pain, sweating day and night, so weak I could not even turn over in bed, let alone get out.

After knocking on my room door, someone said, "Are you in there?"

My weak reply was "yes".

Then through the door I heard "Are you okay?"

With as much effort as I could possibly muster, I replied "no".

And then they came barreling in, headed by the same nurse who, less than two weeks previously, had discounted the bite based on her view from across the counter.

She sat down on the bed next to me, grave concern appeared on her face following her examination of me. Her diagnosis: Lyme.

They were now all gazing over my weak, limp body in the bed. Within a week and a half I had been taken down by this meningitis fever which nearly killed me. I sweated it out in pain for three days, alone and unable to get out of bed or call for help.

In the few extremely brief, feverish conscious moments I did have during the three day ordeal, I knew I was in trouble but I had been too weak to get help for myself.

I only remember being conscious a few times. The pain in particular in my neck was horrific and scary. I thought of trying to get out of bed to get help, but I was much too weak. Then, still laying in bed, I would pass out again from the fever and pain, wishing I could call for help as consciousness slipped away.

I lost half my body weight in the process. Later a co-worker told me that I had lost so much weight she didn't even recognize me. She said she was afraid to touch me because I looked so frail.

I wish I could tell you that they got me to the right help right away and that was the end of the disease. But I can't. It actually got worse and was going to get a lot worse as time went on.

Back to the discovery of me in my room. As it was already four o'clock on a Sunday afternoon, they determined it was best to send me to the emergency walk-in clinic. They found a volunteer to drive me in my car up to the walk-in clinic. He promptly left me there saying he did not feel like waiting and drove my car back to campus. Before he left he said I should call a taxi to take me back to campus. I was too sick to argue so he left me there alone, no wallet, no money as he drove himself back to campus in my car. This was all taking place at 4:00 on a Sunday afternoon!

As I sat crouched quietly holding my exploding head in my hands, there was a great ruckus going on in the walk-in clinic waiting room between the other patients. Apparently, one lady had failed to sign-in and was missing her turn. She was angry because she wanted to go to the movies — the other people waiting would not let her jump the line even though they knew she had been there before them. Oh my, I thought to myself 'they cannot be that sick with all this arguing going on…" and I just kept sitting quietly holding my pounding head and rocking in the corner.

Finally the doctor came into the waiting room and shouted "all right, stop this, you will all have to decide between yourselves who will go next!'

All at once the whole room turned around and pointed at me and said "we want *her* to go next!" I was so surprised as I had not said anything to anyone while I was waiting. I just sat quietly in the corner and could only imagine that I obviously looked that sick that they knew I needed help fast.

As I go in to visit with the harried emergency walk-in clinic doctor, I ask *him* if he wants to see the bite on my leg, and *he* says *NO* too!

In total, he spent less than five minutes interviewing me about my symptoms, all without looking at me or touching me. He discounted me just as the three previous medical personnel attendants had. His response to my asking him to look at the bite was "No, I don't need to see the bite. Just take these, and you will be fine," as he ripped a scribbled prescription from his pad. Then, without looking back, he was onto the next impatient patient waiting for his or her share of attention-less care.

From there it was four weeks of doxycycline, which temporarily reduced the crippling symptoms but did not cure the Lyme.

It is useful to note here that once one has been bitten by a tick infected with Lyme disease, the bacteria will live in the bloodstream for eight to eleven days. You have the best chance of eradicating this disease during this time, which is prior to the spirochetes burrowing infestation into drug-free hiding places within the body.

Beyond the eight to eleven days, these Lyme bacteria then take the form of a spiral corkscrew shape called a spirochete. With this formation they then burrow in with a corkscrew motion and drill their way into the bone, cartilage, brain—all places within your body where medication cannot go.

These spirochetes form little cysts to protect themselves from medications and our immune system. The cysts are coated with an impenetrable mucus called biofilm constructed in part from the toxic heavy metals within our body. Heavy metal toxicity comes from the air we breathe, amalgam fillings, and vaccines, aluminum cooking pans — to name a few sources.

Another danger for us while the spirochetes are within their cyst formation is replication. When these cysts burst open, one spirochete has now become seven. This expansion cycle continues, repeatedly birthing spirochetes until there is finally a collapse of the overgrown colony, only to have another group of spirochetes build another biofilm-protected colony somewhere else in the body. These new colonies then expand and then collapse again and again in a vicious cycle of hide and seek.

The Lyme colony growth cycle continues unabated. Toxic bacterial and/or viral waste builds up in the body as a result of the respiration, sweat, and defecation from these spirochete colonies living and dying.

The pain we experience is our inflamed body continually working to clean out toxic debris left when spirochete colonies die off. This is sometimes known as a Herxheimer reaction, or herxing when spoken of in Lyme community support groups and by medical community members.

I took four weeks of the prescribed antibiotic doxycycline. This medication was like a grenade going off in my stomach and ripping my gut apart with every dose I tried to keep down. I have a very weak stomach to begin with, and I do not do well with pharmaceuticals. Both combined were a disaster. I required four weeks off from work to rest while taking the medication. Feeling better, I was able to return to my appreciated position as program coordinator.

Yet within two weeks following the completion of the prescribed antibiotics and my return to work, my symptoms started to flare again. This time it manifested as lower left groin lymph pain with a dull ache coupled with general exhaustion and a low-grade malaise.

As the groin pain grew I tried to ignore the dull ache, not realizing it was a furthering of the disease. At times a wave of illness would surge through me, and I needed to sit or lie down for relief as it progressed. At these times I would look green and pasty. Family members would exclaim,with stressed concern, how ill I looked.

At this time, my attention was again drawn to this bump on the outside of my thigh, still there, the size of a grain of sand. No one had heeded my request to look at what I thought was a tick bite.

I thought to myself, *What is this thing?*

I started working on it and finally decided to dig it out myself. My instinct told me I needed it removed *now*! So I dug and pried ... nothing; it was just there. *But I'm on a mission now,* I thought. *This isn't normal.* Locating the tweezers, I sterilized them and began to gingerly explore.

Now, this thing was really in there. With patience, however, eventually I was successful—it was *out*!

Oh, but now there were new things happening in my body.

This tiny bump was actually the tick that had been burrowed in all this time—eight weeks! With its removal there resulted a puncture wound that bled for at least twenty minutes. Nine years later I still have a keloid scar in that location that can be extremely sensitive at times as it molts.

Now new symptoms were rapidly emerging. The scariest was a pain sensation racing along the right side of my body, up and down from head to toe, like lightening strikes. I began to feel faint, and my heart started beating as if it were going to pound right out of my chest.

The symptoms raged again and again. This time I went to management and revealed the abuse I had experienced at the hands of their medical staff. This particular manager did not like what I had to say and defended the campus medical team. Sicker than ever, not finding support, I finally resigned from a job I loved.

I went back to my cabin and, with the help of God alone, loaded my few possessions into my car and left.

Within a few days of me resigning from my wonderful job, the top official from campus called to check on me, as apparently word had reached him about my situation. I truly appreciated his caring and reaching out. He was supportive and kind and urged me to see any physician I felt comfortable with to be sure I had been effectively treated for Lyme. I thanked him and begged to end the call because my heart was racing so horrifically. I could not stand up straight, and I thought I would have a stroke or something worse right there in the kitchen.

From then on, I was bedridden. I would give it my best to rally at times, to shake this sickness off somehow, but this was something much bigger than I could handle. It had me in the grip of death, and I was never so alone as in the moments and years to follow, save God by my side.

Over the following months and years my struggles included no less than

> a scar from the tick bite still evident today; meningitis fever; bladder infections; hallucinations; bedridden; rashes; neck aches; severe memory loss; pink-eye; ringing in the ear; vertigo; involuntary muscle twitching; arthritic joint pain and weakness;

bell's palsy, feeling like my legs were going to give out when walking; falling down the stairs following a brain seizure; difficulty talking; difficulty driving; feeling as if bugs were crawling under my skin; mood swings; chronic fatigue; deep chest colds and coughs; muscle aches; digestive issues; vomiting; constipation; pain, pain, pain everywhere pain, including the big toe joint, pain similar to gout and headaches so bad I prayed for God to take me; poor eyesight; eye nerve pain; extreme, irrational raging anger; confusion and memory loss.

All the while I was searching for answers. I just kept searching and praying for answers. They came one at a time.

LESSON #2: JUDGMENT IS NOT ALWAYS A BAD THING

I HAVE TO tell you it is hard writing this. It is hard to summon up these details in my memory and print negative commentary. I like to think people are good and try their best in all endeavors in life.

But outrageously I didn't see anyone practicing attention to detail within the medical care system early on in my case. Now that I have recovered enough to talk to other Lyme suffers, both in and out of support groups, I find many of their frustrations and experiences to be similar. This is tragic because they cannot find recovery nor relief from the medical community for Lyme disease with the present protocol as it stands today. They endure and live a life of illness and disability without hope. Each year is more draining than the last.

Many are lost, hurt, confused, shamed, abandoned, and left searching for answers. I am pressing on here for their sake, to give *hope* and impress to keep the *faith*, to let them know they are *not alone* and they are not crazy.

There is an answer. Recovery is absolutely possible.

The most compassionate, helpful, and effective medical professionals I found were those few who have experienced Lyme disease and co-infections themselves.

I recognized a pattern within the main medical community that was attempting to treat me. I realized every medical person I went to seek help from, especially at the time of the bite, all reacted the same way. They basically could not have cared less about the supposed bite, clearly marked on my leg. They did not care about my symptoms. They did not care about early intervention. They did not care about me. They did not want to go beyond the industry-standard ineffective protocol. They basically made me feel like they just wanted me to go away, die, and not bother them. I was repeatedly discounted, humiliated, judged, questioned, and made to feel suspect and wrong for seeking help for such a small incident as a tick bite and the overwhelming disability of Lyme disease that resulted.

During the initial stages of the tick bite, had anyone in the medical community taken the time to apply even the most basic, rudimentary skill of just looking at the tick embedded in my thigh and removing it in a timely manner, up close and personal, this disease and the subsequent *years* of suffering, pain, and loss could have been totally avoided.

Looking back, I remember my intuition signaling judgmental thoughts based on what I thought was the medical attendants lack of attention to details during examinations. It had me doubting their competency but I was too sick to think clearly for my own best good. I blindly trusted those who have sworn to do no harm. Big mistake.

Trying to be fair and not hoist my demanding standards onto others, I assumed everyone else was as interested and blessed in their work as I was. I believed others cared as much for my welfare, in their hands, as I cared for those who came to me for my professional healing therapeutic skills.

I learned I was wrong. I learned the medical community must be approached with a "buyer beware" attitude. Since then I have learned to take my power back. I was forced to find my voice and become my own advocate. Now I employ a greater sense of discernment.

Now I stand in my own truth.

THE HAND OF GOD

IN TAKING MY power back, I gave myself permission to recognize the Hand of God in all of this. Ultimately, I have determined this very act led me to discover the gift of Lyme disease at journeys end.

This happened as I earnestly prayed daily for help. Excellent doctors started to become available. There were three who helped the most and I will always be indebted to them for their compassion and skill. One was my chiropractor, who was indispensable. The next was a wonderful psychiatrist who herself had battled Lyme disease for years and suffered greatly. The third was a former IDSA doctor who recognized chronic Lyme and bravely worked to answer the clarion call for help.

God fed me through my daily struggle. As I surrendered to the journey by aligning with health laws in the Bible, I got stronger. Regaining my health was hard won, but worth the getting.

"One finger pointing out, three fingers pointing back" is a familiar saying.

One day I looked at my hand mimicking this posture as I counted up all the medical people who brushed away the initial tick bite. As my counting took up every finger, I realized it was indeed the hand of God in action. No one person was to blame, it was many. It was this very hand that for years sculpted, kneaded, thumped, tugged, and rubbed in the honored role of body worker, licensed massage therapist, and energy healer which was now, itself, reaching out for help.

To me, my role as healer is an honor bestowed upon me by the earned trust from clients who enter a vulnerable, sacred space and allow healing to take place. I have spent years traveling around the world and spent countless hours continually studying, training, and refining my craft to be the best that I can be.

And again, I just assumed others were consciously following their bliss. Like myself, especially here at this wonderful place of enlightenment. Painfully, I discovered this is not entirely true at all.

As the years of dealing with Lyme mounted and the pain wracked my body with an ugly, dark and indescribable tearing, I prayed for God to take me.

I wanted someone to blame. *Yes, it must be someones fault!* I was sure of it. Only the echo of "one finger pointing out, three pointing back" kept me focused on the fact that I could solve this problem with time.

God did not and would not abandon me.

I knew better then to think of myself as a victim. And another great truth is the fact that 'Blame takes the focus off of you'.

God had given me an assignment. Yes, I recognized the signs all too well.

The journey embarked upon was not to be along a strait and narrow road but, rather, a wandering, circuitous route and not for the faint of heart.

I felt all but abandoned by most of the medical community who could only offer temporary antibiotic fixes with no good answer. I finally took matters into my own hands and designed a kitchen-cabinet cure incorporating botanicals from Mother Nature's traditional common-sense wisdom.

Mother Nature will respond at the ready when trouble strikes. The cure appears along with the disease. With this burgeoning Lyme epidemic Mother Nature has brought in invasive weeds to save the day.

Looking back, I can see now what I could not see then. The wheels were clearly off the cart and I was speeding downhill fast and all alone. As I continued the Lyme healing journey, I found this same painfully discouraging attitude over and over again from within the medical community.

Sadly, I see the reports of over 300,000 newly diagnosed cases of Lyme per year, and that is not counting the misdiagnosed cases, that plague our medical community. All sufferers, properly diagnosed or not, are left searching for answers for recovery and relief.

As my disease burrowed in deeper, it turned into Chronic Neurological Lyme, which landed me in bed for five years. I was to see no fewer than fifteen doctors and ultimately received a written prognosis stating I would never work again.

I actually experienced hallucinations during the depths of this disease. I was terrified and very alone. Everything looked hopeless.

I eventually found there is an answer. There is a natural and safe way to go about healing all of this. It is simple but not always easy. This is why we are here.

This chronic illness lasting for years helped me find out who my friends really were. I cherish them today. I lost most of them as time dragged on. They wondered why I was not getting over it. Gone from sight, forgotten from the heart.

No longer able to sustain the athletic prowess of a high-functioning, full-time veteran massage therapist, I had to close my healing practice. This was a devastating blow. Most of my clients had been with me since I opened and they were wonderful and kind. I was no longer able to be self-employed in the profession that I loved and had trained my entire focus on for years. Nor was I employable for even the most basic jobs outside that arena.

On and off antibiotics. In and out of no fewer than fifteen doctors offices. Off meds, sick. On meds, still sick, barely able to function. Then off again and sicker still. Now I was homeless and jobless, unemployable. There was no relief. There were times, too, that I endured disgusted looks from frustrated people who did not understand why I was not already better.

I searched for answers in the alternative world where I am most comfortable and began to find clues to a cure. As I worked with these tools I began to see very slow progress. I am writing my story of recovery to explain my experience with the hope that there may be an answer for you here.

There is a gift with Lyme disease at journeys end. It is worth it. Keep the faith. Now I am back to work and in love with life again. As a result of all of this I have dedicated my life to helping others with chronic Lyme and co-infections. Together we are breaking through to new and better levels of personal health and vitality.

It is not easy. People are sick, scared, and afraid to incorporate natural cleansing and detoxing tools, which for me were keys for resourcing rejuvenation. Forbidden topics — when we say the word *colonics* or *enemas*! People flee the room left and right! But this therapy is very beneficial since 80 percent of our immune system is in our gut. It is said all disease starts in the gut.

Since my recovery from chronic neurological Lyme disease, many people I have spoken with regarding Lyme have had their appendixes out. For me that was a fleeting fear. When I felt a sharp, stabbing pain in my appendix region, I got right on the colonic bed regularly. Prior to Lyme I had only been receiving professional colonics occasionally over the years with excellent results. This therapy is well worth the cost. As I worked to overcome my Lyme disability, I discovered cost-saving at-home enemas to be even more highly beneficial in developing a clearer and truer relationship with my body, its needs and the language it communicates with.

Now I absolutely shine! I have the bounce back in my step. I am happier and healthier then I have been in years. I know who I am. I took my power back, and I did the work. We are a special tribe, those of us who work to overcome this horrific disease.

Much more went into my recovery, but perhaps we are starting to get a little bit ahead of ourselves.

God Bless you all for taking this enormous journey.

SURRENDER

YES, I SAID it. I know it may feel completely counter-intuitive. We think we want to bomb, nuke, and annihilate the bugs! We are fighting for our lives!

You are not alone. We have heard science tell us we are composed of 90 percent microbes—germs! They thrive throughout our bodies trillions of cells, located in the digestive tract, skin, organs, mouth, nose, and ears!

Lyme disease disability provided the tension necessary to do the work of conscious development.

It provided the propulsion mechanism for personal evolution and growth.

Lyme taught me who I was deep down inside. I had to get right with God (fill in your name for the Universal Life Source). I recognized the need to surrender to this situation and go from there.

Lyme has a gift, whereby, you will finally claim your vibrational liquid luminescent light body. Recovery is re-sourcing our joyous, amazing focus into alignment with these health and wellness principals which bring us peace, love and tranquility.

This journey has a higher purpose of discovering more intently our zero balance point between wisdom and compassion. I reviewed and shifted everything relating to my lifestyle and nutrition. Everything received a tilling and a turning, over and over, for proper review. You will grow, dear one. All will be well.

The first step to holistically healing acute states of chronic illness is to shift your mindset to one of surrender. Many people think they know what surrender is. Reactions to this concept range from anger to curiosity to comprehension. How do we surrender? If we say "I have turned it over" one time, does this does not create true surrender? No, it is not enough.

According to the Merriam-Webster Dictionary, the definition of surrender is:

noun
: an agreement to stop fighting, hiding, resisting, etc., because you know that you will not win or succeed : an act of surrendering
: the act of giving the control or use of something to someone else
: the act of allowing yourself to be influenced or controlled by someone or something

transitive verb
a : to yield to the power, control, or possession of another upon compulsion or demand <*surrendered* the fort>

b : to give (oneself) over to something (as an influence)

I like transitive verb b definition listed above: to give (oneself) over to something (as an influence). That influence was my belief that the body has an inner wisdom which does the healing. When we surrender are we saying we are giving up? Are we quitting? Does Lyme win?

No! We are just putting down the weapons of warfare and creating a compassionate strategy in this game of life.

So, what does a surrender mindset look like? Why would we need to surrender? How does one completely surrender? What are the benefits? Who or what are we surrendering to?

Surrender, for someone healing from a chronic illness, is a state of being in a heart-centered space where there is no blame, no anger, and no war. It shifts into an adventure of skill and leadership in the search to find the zero point balance between wisdom and compassion which is centered entirely around love.

—Suzen

It is simply comprehending life as the unfolding of the consequences of our actions. It is not good nor bad. It just *is*. We are just one component of the complex, cosmic whole.

When I first got sick I wanted to blame all four medical personnel I encountered during the first two weeks of my illness for not doing what they could have to prevent my illness from progressing. Make no mistake about it: Lyme disease for me at that time could have been totally prevented. I did all the right things. I asked all four medical people to look at the bite in a timely manner as I had been instructed, but no one seemed to care. Two medical attendants each glanced at the bite from afar and dismissed it. The third told me my fever, along with pain in my occiput and sacrum, was a cold. The fourth was the emergency room doctor who did not want to look at the bite as he wrote the prescription saying, "Just take this for four weeks, and you'll be fine." I did as he instructed, and I wasn't.

Ultimately, I understood I gave my power away. I ignored my gut instinct over and over again. The only way for me to fully recover would be for me to take back my power and practice self-responsibility, right up to and including, all the vibrational manifestations from my own thought processes.

I finally realized that even though my three outstanding doctors were doing their best with full knowledge of the difficulties I faced, I needed to take matters into my own hands. I knew these good doctors cared deeply, that was clear. But I began to recognize I needed to explore beyond what these doctors were presenting as options. I needed to step-up and show-up in a bigger way no matter what it took.

I set about to devise a new plan, a new mindset. But what would that be? This disease nearly killed me. The court-ordered doctors report said I would never work again. How could this be happening? I had been completely healthy and happy before this tick bite—everything was fine! Now my life was in ruins, and I was desperate for answers.

At a certain point I began to think of this as a fight for my life. My inflamed, raging mindset was fierce, and I was going to win at any cost against this dastardly foe called Lyme!

I had to continually remind myself to surrender. It was not war. It actually required strategy. Turn it over, and over and over, every time, my incoherent mind raged, I reminded myself to regroup and think strategically.

FIGHT FOR YOUR LIFE AND THE ART OF WAR

WHEN AN ANGEL whispered in my ear with a message that such an angry and aggressive attitude was not the answer, I immediately surrendered. Such negative energy was only creating bitter resentment, rage, and anxiety, causing an acidic inner terrain that blocked my divine healing vibrational capability.

> In times of peace, sons bury fathers;
>
> In times of war, fathers bury sons.

From my years of healing work as a licensed massage therapist I knew the angels messages were right. It made total sense.

From then on, conscious prayer and meditation on a regular basis permanently shifted this mindset. Once these tools were in place I was able to manage the chronic pain a bit more, which gave me great hope that I was on the right path.

One of the later symptoms of Lyme was the development of what I came to describe as a pox-mark-like rash on my legs, arms, shoulders, neck, and face. These would start out as little parchment puffs of white, delicate skin. As I instinctively touched them I would rub them off as one would rub off dry skin. Then underneath that spot I would immediately develop a round splotch of bloody skin. It would bleed and scab over. This scab would last for many, many weeks. As I am fair-skinned, these marks really stood out, and no amount of cover-up makeup would send these disgusting signs of deep disease into the nether regions and allow me to pretend I was fit to move about society. I felt like I had the walking plague from the Middle Ages.

Then I had another awakening as to a better, more natural healing tool. A vision came to me about embracing this new, peaceful strategy. Remembering when as children my siblings and I had chicken pox, I had a vision of my Dad cooking up brown soap that he shaved into a pot of hot water and melted into a paste. He then proceeded to slather this brown goo on our pox-marked bodies as we all lined up in the living room. It was yucky but it did the trick to soothe and heal our itchy bodies. My Lyme pox marks were not itchy but this vision reminded me there was a natural way to deal with illness.

The next vision was yet another time involving my Dad. This time he was teaching me to play chess, a game of strategy. We were in the same spot in the living room where a few years earlier he had treated our chicken pox with the brown soap paste.

Now I was to remember the importance of strategic thinking as taught to me by my Dad while playing chess.

I began to appreciate that these bacterial colonies are an essential force of nature with their own purpose for existence. They too desire survival, just as all other living organisms in God's creative world who propel themselves perpetually toward survival.

These Lyme spirochetes were not out to purposely hurt me. It was not personal. Lyme was just being its bacterial true self and had as much right to exist as any other creature in God's creation. I just desired this not to be at the cost of my health please!

I decided to no longer wage a violent war within my body against these spirochetes but rather to orchestrate a peaceful surrender for the spirochetes. I decided they would have a final day to choose to stay or go. They would go according to my timing, by the action of me putting my personal wellness front and center.

Continuing on with this developmental strategy, I also remembered a term called 'red-lining' from my studies in Public Policy at Trinity College regarding inner-city crime. Law enforcement officials knew they could never get rid of crime. The goal was instead to create a strategy of containment called 'red-lining' where the focus was to corral crime into certain sections of the city. This would allow law enforcement to more easily coordinate forces to contain and manage crime within these directed areas and thereby preventing rampant spread of criminal entities beyond these limits. Lyme would now be Red Lined.

So I made Lyme disease and co-infections my opponent in a game of chess and devised a strategy to win at this game of life. I set out to learn all I could about Lyme's habits—what it ate and drank, eliminated, how it slept, reproduced, and died; the structure of its society; and its defenses, communication abilities, and purpose in nature.

I worked to maneuver and manipulate my inner terrain and internal playing field to my advantage. My goal was to claim back my inner territory and eliminate Lyme one spirochete at a time. It was a fact that I had to get every single spirochete, for if even one was left, the disease would again rage within.

Developing my ability to navigate the Internet for research became invaluable as I pursued healthy healing tools. I could only venture online for moments at a time in the beginning; as I would do research online sitting at my laptop computer.

The cosmic giggle appeared as I discovered electromagnetic fields (EMFs) actually feed the spirochetes. Therefore, the greater my online research time on the laptop, the greater the painful herxing experience.

Most of my ill Lyme years I would consider to have been one big Herx. The term *herxing* is used to describe the pain when spirochete colonies collapse. The pain that follows is the result of the body's efforts to clean up the colonies gaseous and metabolic debris.

With these herxing episodes I would continually end up in bed for a week to ten days following my online computer searches. As I recovered from each explosive herxing episode, I would again venture back online for more research, and the cycle would play out over and over again.

More research followed by more pain for days, months, and years on end. I was prisoner to these dominating episodes until I discovered the connection between EMF exposure and the colony growth expansion which always flared following my online computer searches.

Perseverance in research revealed the answer to managing the EMF exposure and herxing cycle was, in fact, to start grounding my body. One simple way is to stand barefoot on the earth or natural stone. It will not work by standing on pavement or cement; our body must be connected directly to the earth.

This facilitates an alignment of negative ions in the body similar to clearing the static from the body that causes an electrical shock when touching a doorknob. I went the extra mile and purchased a kit containing a cotton bed sheet with silver threads running through it. This sheet attaches to the grounding plug in the wall by a cord attached to the silver-threaded sheet. By this method I was grounded all night as I slept.

For months before grounding myself, the pain at the bottom of my feet had increased and made walking nearly impossible, especially upon rising in the morning. It was so bad at one point I could not place my bare feet on the floor without excruciatingly sharp pains consuming the bottom of my feet.

Additionally arthritic pain riddled my body in the joints, soft tissue, just everywhere. Once I started sleeping on the grounding sheet and standing outside barefoot—even in the winter—I awoke in the morning pain free. It was absolutely amazing.

Another tool in the grounding kit is a rubber grounding pad which I keep on my desktop as I work on the computer. This rubber pad is also attached to the grounding port in the wall with a cord. As I am working on the computer with waves of EMFs continually being emitted at me, I am grounded and the charge drains off me when I am touching the grounded rubber pad. Such a blessing provided much relief.

As I made these step-by-step connections, I would tackle each problem and incorporate that change into my daily lifestyle habits and routine. These steps were simple but not always easy. To create a new habit takes 21 to 40 days of repeating the desired action before it becomes truly second nature.

Pain is a great motivator. I had no problem using these tools and seeing slow but recognizable results. My consistent research efforts began to pay off, yielding more vital clues.

One such monumental discovery was that Lyme hides in the roots of teeth that have been filled. It turns out that once a tooth has had its integrity compromised with a filling, the tooth loses its natural ability to cleanse bacteria from itself. Therefore, these teeth have been found to be a perfect breeding ground for Lyme and co-infection bacteria.

Necrotic tissue resulting from root canals are even more deadly. All the tiny channels beyond the main root system are so small they cannot be filled like the main root channel. These smaller capillary-like channels become perfect hiding and breeding spots for the spirochetes. These hollow chambers are warm and moist, and they expel the breeding spirochetes each time one bites down.

Discovering the fact that Lyme hides in the teeth presented me with my next goal, which was to remove mercury fillings along with my gold crown tooth. During the removal, my dentist discovered the gold crown was actually mixed metals and acted like a battery imbedded in my jaw tissue. Add the necrotic tissue from the root canal that is left behind in dentistry, and there you have another favorite place for spirochetes to hide and breed.

The crown component damaged my jaw tissue so extensively as to require a two-stage procedure. One year the crown was removed. I then had to wait for another year while the tissue healed to be well enough to sustain the seriously aggressive surgical removal of the root canal stub, along with all surrounding necrotic tissue.

The second stage of removing the root canal stub was overwhelming because they actually had to scrape much of the jawbone away to clean up the damaged tissue. It was so serious the dentist called that evening to check on my recovery process. Just remembering that single procedure still gives me chills today. But it worked and I'm worth it!

When I suggest this important step to clients or people who are seeking advice on recovering from Lyme, I get a lot of naysayers. They stumble over the cost, the time, the pain.

I too had to weigh very carefully the option of investing significant funds into all of these procedures. I also needed a car, a place to live, day-to-day living expenses, and the like. And I could not work.

My quandary was painfully obvious but I really had only one answer relying on one theory: fix the teeth; which would fix the health; which would fix the income; which would fix the other problems.

Once I bravely took the steps for healing into my own hands, my healing began to turn a corner. I placed my faith in God, knowing all would be well even though I could not see how at that time.

Removing the amalgam fillings along with a mixed-metal crown and necrotic root canal tissue was equivalent to removing an iron mask from my head. The relief was so significant I would recommend these dental procedures while one is still in good health!

Healing still progressed slowly but again it was another step forward toward regaining my health. These are important procedures for everyone to consider.

Following the successful dental work I continued doing the next thing in front of me and then the next thing and then the next. Slowly, slowly, ever so slowly, enough progress was made to eventually get me back on my feet and beat this diagnosis of permanent disability. I would not give up, ever.

Continual perseverance revealed many more tools to help boost my immune system, which resulted in what I have come to affectionately call the most cost-effective kitchen-cabinet cures. No longer counting on professional medical intervention and instead choosing traditional, herbal, natural cures from Mother Nature herself, I was able to sustain increasing wellness with growing stamina.

Here is a very important element to remember:

> *You can know all the right things to do,*
> *but if you do not do them in the right order,*
> *they will not work!*

MINDSET—JUST THE FACTS

CHECKMATE! I *WIN!*

Everything counts. Get clear on the facts. It is a daily struggle to keep aligned with goodness and positive healing thoughts when feeling so ill. Keeping things in the right order means dealing with our mindset and thought patterns in the present time. Subconscious issues can throw us off track, especially when we are drained from battling a chronic illness as devastating as Lyme disease and co-infections.

Of course this must be done a little at a time. The way to move a mountain is a pebble at a time. Stress and frustration can easily derail our efforts. Daily focus on your healthy goals and overall lifestyle habits is priceless.

Know the facts when dealing with Lyme, but do not get caught up in the politics of the conspiracy theory. Channel your energy toward healing your own body. It matters not that Lyme disease may have been engineered on Plum Island. The fact is you have it now; deal with it here and now. After you recover you can take up that cause if you feel the need, but for now, it is a moot point.

Know what to call it! This disease was named for Lyme, Connecticut, where the first case was diagnosed. One doctor yelled at me because I was confused about the name. I heard people use both "Lyme" and "Lyme's" and refer to themselves as "Lymies". I started using both "Lyme" and "Lymes" interchangeably when referencing the disease in conversation. One day I nearly cried as a doctor yelled at me. "It's *Lyme*, not *Lymes*!" came barreling through the telephone into my already sensitive ear.

This fact drove home the importance of needing to correctly identify the opponent I was dealing with on every level. You cannot hit a target if the mark is off.

Furthermore, please do not fall into the habit of calling it "*my* Lyme" or call yourself a "Lymie". This opens the door to enmeshment with disease on a subconscious and energetic level. You are not your disease! You are a host. You will experience a big difference in healing results.

More confusion along with some clarity: it is a bacteria, it is a virus! It has been classified as one or the other over the years. It replicates and feeds on sugar, processed foods, nightshade vegetables, stress hormones, chronic acidosis, heavy metals, and a toxic lifestyle. Lyme disease and co-infections are opportunistic parasites sucking your life force and polluting your inner ecosystem with their off-gassing excrement and metabolic waste. We must make sure our channels of elimination are working well so that we have minimal toxic exposure buildup.

Lyme has been around for ages. Testing of the remains from the ice-age man revealed he had been afflicted with Lyme. This fact gave me comfort and confirmation of nature at work. I began to refer to Lyme as just a misplaced bacteria, now within me.

The secret focus was to make my inner terrain inhospitable to Lyme disease and co-infections. That meant getting alkaline and that meant addressing my lymphatic system along with improving kidney filtration and adrenal output.

Our lymphatic system is our garbage disposal specifically designed to remove metabolic waste, cancer, parasites, viruses, bacteria, heavy metals, pesticides, fluoride, BPA, vaccines, pharmaceuticals and more. When this system is sluggish and backed up from a sedentary lifestyle, we poison ourselves from the inside out.

Another small sidebar fact that made a difference for me was when I learned that the true nature of spirochetes is to spawn the growth of deer antlers. Obviously, we do not have antlers, but it is fascinating to note Lyme has a purpose in nature. The spirochetes use their continual spiraling action of ascension to gain access into our bodies deepest regions. Perhaps to mimic their function within deer antlers and facilitating the antlers growth.

My experience with medical science is they are missing this major sticking point in connection with how to coax these spirochetes out of these hiding places. Tinctures of Teasel Root, Japanese Knotweed, Andrographis and flower essences are the most essentially useful tools for these problematic stumbling blocks, in a complete healing recovery journey from Lyme.

Most favored is Teasel root, which coaxes spirochetes out of protective hiding places. Next we are blessed with Japanese knotweed which is loaded with Resveratrol and is a natural antibiotic all at the same time. Two common invasive roadside plants which are found to behave powerfully in overcoming Lyme disease. Andrographis is wonderful as a preventative tincture which I now use whenever I have been out working in the garden and possibly exposed to ticks.

In alchemy the "poison is the cure". Mother Nature confidently provides all we need.

MIND YOUR MIRROR

MINDSET IS THE capstone that supports our complex structure of reality. Our thoughts manifest our reality. Now we address the question of healing considering the role of genetics vs epi-genetics. In genetics we believe we will face the same fate as our fore-family. According to Bruce Lipton, author of Biology of Belief, he states that within epi-genetics we comprehend a higher thought pattern and reasoning. By creating a newer healthier vision, whereby we facilitate our ability to over-ride our genetic predisposition, we are able to change our healing destiny. Just because our family lineage suffered certain diseases does not mean our fate is sealed. But we must be diligent in keeping our thoughts positive and pure through meditation and spiritual belief.

When addressing spiritual beliefs I am not saying religious beliefs, they are two different concepts. Spiritually speaking we have direct access to Universal source which is loving and compassionate. Religious beliefs require an intermediary such as a priest to pray for our intercession. Religion can be punitive and restrictive. Spirituality puts us in a position of direct responsibility for acting with love and compassion in all that we do. You are not entrapped by your family lineage and doomed to suffer just as your ancestors did. With spiritual beliefs you are in charge and can break the chains that bind. It is a journey where you realize All is One. What you do to another, you do to yourself. Consequences of your actions yield either negative or positive results. Spirituality is a much broader field of vision which challenges our soul in a different way. This is the way into changing your genetic destiny. This is the way of healing.

When we apply spiritual love and compassion to our Lyme healing journey, it is no longer acceptable to introduce mass destruction with an overload of antibiotics which wipe out beneficial gut flora along with the bad. This will put our future health in jeopardy.

The lifecycle of the Lyme spirochetes involves free-flowing bacteria circulating within our bloodstream. From the bloodstream these bacterial spirochete corkscrew deeper into our bones, cartilage, brain, and organs—basically, all the best and safest hiding and breeding places.

These hiding places are previously weakened areas within our body which have become acidic through either physical or emotional trauma. The longer Lyme is allowed to run free and nestle into each of these inappropriately acidic areas, the more damage it leaves behind and the more difficult it is to eradicate. If the invasive infection is contained early, there is a greater chance of successful recovery.

For some this journey is also a path of awakening and a journey into ones very soul. This is where we apply our loving, compassionate, spiritually healing beliefs. Change your thoughts, change your belief, change your destiny. Forgiveness, Love and Compassion lead the way.

OUTSMART THE BUGGERS BEFORE THEY OUTSMART YOU

SO, IF LYME spirochetes have always been in existence within our body throughout history, this brings the question: what exactly has changed with our relationship to Lyme, that now it is at epidemic proportions running rampant in the general population?

Many authorities today point to our growing exposure to dirty electricity. This new and disruptive energetic vibration is seriously affecting our inner terrain and forcing it out of harmony with our previous ancient rhythm with the spirochetes, whereby, we could keep them in check. Perhaps it is something to consider which might be a great contributing factor in the widening of this Lyme epidemic.

Our pain is pointing us toward imbalances in our lives which need immediate attention. There is no pain where there is no problem. There is no denying the pain of Lyme when it has the upper hand in our body.

Record keeping becomes important in relation to understanding the timing of colony bloom and collapse and the resulting herxing episodes. Through regular journaling I could see which of my lifestyle habits brought about good and bad results. Tracking foods eaten to identify any resulting pain patterns provided evidence by revealing the foods and lifestyle habits which were feeding or not feeding the Lyme colonies. This colony bio-film die-off requires our body to take on the extra load of cleaning up their cellular debris and toxins, thereafter, resulting in herxing inflammatory pain. Some contributing factors to continued colony growth are EMF exposure, heavy metals, biofilm strength, poor nutrition, anxiety, and stress.

When self-treating we can outsmart these little buggers with a slight shift and change-up of supplement and tincture schedules. They have their own intelligent life force which enables them to work and communicate together within their own communities. This knitting together of their life force shield facilitates their instinctive thriving and survival intentions which allows them to predict just when medications will be dispensed into their environment. By catching them off guard, we have a better chance of preventing their instinctive return to their safe haven.

Throughout all of these healing crises and experiences I observed these secrets that the medical community was overlooking and not incorporating. These major elemental secrets of how to get the spirochetes out of these hiding places, along with using Mother Nature's natural antibiotic, plus an improved correct mindset and clean living, all work together to bring us back into balance. These insights provided the key advantage. Once I enacted specific strategies addressing these details, I upped my game of recovery quite a bit more. My intention when using all tools was "game over" for Lyme and its co-infection friends.

This is a "simple" but not "easy" protocol as we turn to Mother Nature for her alchemical solution for relief.

YOU CAN KNOW ALL THE RIGHT THINGS TO DO ... BUT IF YOU DO NOT DO THEM IN THE RIGHT ORDER, THEY WILL NOT WORK

DENTAL CARE IS one of the most important items to have in the right order.

As discussed earlier, once a tooth has been drilled and filled, it looses the ability to naturally clean out bacterial and viral metabolic waste. Without this regular cleansing activity of the surrounding intra-cellular environment, we are trapped in a downward spiral leading to painful inflammation. The root canal stump left behind is necrotic tissue and interwoven with many tiny capillary root-canals, which form a network well beyond the original main root-canal extracted. These small canals are perfect dark breeding grounds for Lyme spirochetes. Add to that heavy-metal amalgam fillings, and there is a perfect brew-pot for this disabling chronic disease.

Next, our nutritional intake needs a thorough review. Stop the ingestion of toxins. No more sugar, fried foods, over-cooked foods, caffeine, alcohol. Calm the inflammation raging throughout the body. An alkaline diet and lifestyle will calm such inflammation within our inner terrain. Eating for blood types O, A, B, or AB provided supportive foods while diminishing the negative food intake impact. The other diets were Body Ecology and Paleo which were wonderfully supportive nutritional systems each.

Simple meals are best. Organic leafy greens, fresh juices, and low glycemic fruits, berries and melons provide wonderful nourishment. High-quality fats, increased hydration, and fermented foods help reset the digestive system probiotic supply.

Experiment with protein, and always make sure it is grass-fed and free-range. Eliminate processed foods, trans-fats, sugars, and carbohydrates. Grains can be controversial for causing Irritable Bowel Syndrome (IBS) symptoms. Dairy is also a mucus-forming irritant that many find relief from by not consuming.

Food combining can reduce digestive stress with these simple rules:

1) Combine protein with veggies—no starch.
2) Combine veggies with starch—no protein.
3) Do not combine protein and starch.

Spiritual nutrition is a vital component of healing. Love and forgiveness are essential. In Quantum healing we start at Zero Point which is Gratitude.

Whenever you find yourself drowning in fear based thoughts, switch to thoughts of gratitude and love. Fear and Faith are two sides of one coin. Both cannot exist at the same time. You are either in Fear or in Faith.

Some may argue that both can exist at the same time. But if you understand Quantum healing, Zero Point healing and nano-particles you will further realize that if you are feeling both at the same time you are not at the Zero Point yet. You are still in the chaos of these energies changing up.

Fear is excitement without the breath.

When dealing with a health crisis such as Lyme, full healing and recovery necessitates you absolutely reach bottom of the barrel fear and then you will experience an initial rush when you fully immerse yourself in gratitude.

If gratitude is a new feeling for you, it may take a moment to recognize the calm state it brings along with it after this rush. That is what you are going for, a calm feeling, even if it is fleeting, you will begin to recognize the difference between fear and Faith. Calm, Strong and Unshakeable. The more you focus in on it, the easier it will be to maintain that state.

Our thoughts emit chemicals in the body, and our cells become accustomed to these chemicals. The more we repeatedly grind down on a thought or habit, the more engrained it becomes in our nervous system. We attract what we think about over and over. As we go through life, our cells call for this chemical bath over and over.

Always come back to Zero Point Quantum Healing Gratitude and Love. 432 Hz is the God vibration of our Heart and the musical note C. Music heals our hearts so enjoy listening to Bach's "Cello Suite No. 1 in G major."

To accommodate this hormonal cellular thirst, we subconsciously set up scenarios in our lives designed to give us that charge. These negative dramatic episodes drain our vital core energy long after an event has happened.

Hanging onto resentment and revenge is like drinking poison and hoping the other person will die from it. Forgiveness is not saying what the person did was right. It is, rather, losing the desire for revenge.

There is a great letting go with Lyme. Really, letting it all go. The drama, the strife, the he-said she-said endless looping — out. Put your health regime first—body, mind, and soul. Accept that all that has happened to this point was for your spiritual development. Let's make some lemonade from our lemons shall we!

During the Lyme healing journey you will experience a tracing back through memories which will reveal keys to unlocking the heart of forgiveness and allowing compassion to replace bitterness. This is all part of the recovery from Lyme. It is a review and a shift as we sort through body-talk pain issues arising from Lyme.

Next up we address our digestive issues. Our bodies contains two fluids: blood and lymph. Spirit resides in the blood which circulates with the pumping of our hearts to deliver nutrients and oxygen throughout the body for cellular metabolism. Lymph, which removes waste from the body, is like a sewage system. It moves through a one-way channel that can be stimulated with gentle bouncing up and down movements. Both fluids and corresponding organs will benefit from being cleaned and detoxed as needed. Blood relates to Liver/Gallbladder and Lymph relates to the Kidneys/Bladder.

Colon cleansing is also essential to rest, heal and reboot our digestive system. Liver and gallbladder cleanses allow the body to properly detox in a timely manner. With these organs clean and functioning properly, the body will have clean blood to circulate in an alkaline state.

Disease has its base in chronic acidosis, which is addressed with lymph and kidney cleansing. A detox to clean the blood will take about three to seven days. Cleaning lymph takes a much longer time, a minimum of a three-month period is even more important for optimal body function.

As we clean up the baser foundational functions of the body, we are able to benefit from the finer vibratory healing tools from Mother Nature. In the Quantum field everything in life vibrates. Flowers and plants which are used for tinctures and herbal remedies all have their own delicate but powerful vibration. Pharmaceuticals, over-the-counter medications, fluoride, mercury, lead, chlorine and more, all have a lower, denser, darker vibration. When one is taking pharmaceuticals, over-the-counter medications, or fluoride in their toothpaste and public tap water, for example, these low-level vibrations cancel the useful, delicate, lighter vibrations of Mother Nature's remedy solutions through this disharmony.

Incorporating Dr. Li Qing Yun (1677–1933) a Chinese medicine physician "Rules for Longevity" aided me in discerning which lifestyle actions to take and which to leave.

1) Do not overeat.
2) Economize thinking and speaking in order to nurture Qi.
3) Minimize your desires.

4) Be modest and do not seek the attention of others. This protects the heart.

5) Protect the body from cold and wind.

6) Do not overindulge in cold drinks; they weaken digestive energy.

7) Refrain from eating too much salt; it can damage the kidneys.

8) Keep serene and quiet in the face of life's changes, and keep the natural laws.

I also spent much time remembering Corinthians 13:4-7:

> Love is Patient, Love is Kind.
> It does not envy, it does not boast, it is not proud.
> It does not dishonor others, it is not self-seeking, it is not easily angered, it keeps no record of wrongs.
> Love does not delight in evil but rejoices with the Truth.
> It always protects, always trusts, always hopes, always perseveres.
> Corinthians 13:4-7

As time goes on and you systematically implement health strategies, the spirochete populations decrease, the body becomes cleaner and stronger. With this population decrease, so too goes the painful inflammation and difficulty of day-to-day living. Happiness and joy will return. Creative solutions to these problems make this happen.

It works! With persistence and a relentless can-do attitude, I overcame this disease, and today I have my sparkling health back. Incorporating these new empowering lifestyle habits into my daily routine, still today, keeps me balanced and feeling excellent. When I do occasionally stray from these guidelines and tools, I do become imbalanced and overall more sensitive to what is going on around me.

Thankfully I have never gone back to the indescribable level of daily pain and despair I experienced while living with active chronic neurological Lyme disease and co-infections. At best living with that disease was a poor excuse for existence, just getting by without hope or joy. Those days are over. Praise God!

CHOOSING THE RIGHT ACTION PLAN

DEVELOP AN ACTION plan based on your present focus from where you are now on your journey. Then write an action plan focus for what you want your life to look like one year from now. Work on at least one health tool per day to move your health status forward. I find that a gentler, but more consistent longer-term protocol is overall more effective, than a harsh, full-force, quick, short-term approach.

Lyme visits every physical, emotional, and spiritual trauma you have ever had and nestles in. Be ready to revisit, review, and renew. As the body begins to let go of these trapped emotional cysts from deep within the body, you may experience what is known as a healing crisis. You may feel more intense sickness as the body expels these previously trapped toxins.

As your body becomes a clearer and more alkaline vessel, you will experience these episodes less dramatically. Also the more emotional baggage you can let go of during these times of purging, the happier, healthier and lighter you will be going forward. For example, while I was having Lyme related intense bladder infection issues, I started using Marshmallow Root and examining what I was 'pissed off' about. As I worked through these issues I realized one day my bladder issues were resolved.

Remember you will most likely go through a healing crisis which may scare you and you may think something is wrong and you may want to stop the healing efforts. This healing crisis is a sign that you are on the right path. You may vomit, have loose stools, runny nose, wax in your ears, rashes, gunk in your eyes. These are all signs that your body is ridding itself of toxins as you administer your healing protocols.

Armed with the official doctors report ordered by the insurance company and provided to the courts for the judges review, it said I would never work again, and yes, I felt that was true. At the rate this disease was growing inside of me and taking me down, I did not think I would make it. But I have always had an inner knowing and I was bound and determined to find a way out of this crisis.

For several years I prayed for God to take me. The days when I prayed for God to take me, I was giving up because the extreme pain was so relentless. I was really suffering during these years. Life was one big Herx! I was very scared, confused, and struggling.

I had gone from being a high-functioning, athletic, self-employed massage therapist; happy mom; and happy volunteer to a withered, non-functioning, babbling, unemployable, seemingly defeated, dependent mess. In a heartbeat it seemed I had lost everything and became vulnerable to the slightest environmental insult.

Only a handful of doctors had true compassion and comprehension about what I was going through. All the other doctors were letting me down left and right.

One even looked at my three positive blood tests and exclaimed he did not believe them. He told me he wanted me to take one of his own tests to be sure of my condition. He wanted to have his lab run the tests. That was fine with me.

For clarity, when this new doctor decided to do his own test to be sure I had Lyme, I took yet another test to appease him. His lab produced my fourth positive test for Lyme.

Shockingly, he decided he did not even believe his own lab test after the results came back positive for Lyme.

So when his own lab test came back with a positive reading, confirming that the prior three tests from my other doctors offices and labs were correct, he sat right across from me, looked me right in the eye, and declared:

"You don't have Lyme disease. In fact, I don't think you ever had Lyme disease."

Sitting there frozen, trying to comprehend through my mental Lyme fog what he was telling me, I could not even react.

Let's review this situation. Here was a doctor, sworn and certified, selected by my insurance company for me to see. I arrived with three positive blood tests for Lyme from three different time periods and three different doctors. In fact I had never had one negative test. My first IDSA doctor's test was so sensitive it also confirmed that this was my first experience with Lyme.

Also a reminder that Lyme is often misdiagnosed as ADHD, ALS, chronic fatigue, fibromyalgia, Parkinson and more. Recently in the news we heard the terrible story of Kris Kristofferson's misdiagnosis of Lyme disease as Alzheimers and they were treating him with Alzheimers medications. Once they corrected the diagnosis and took him off the Alzheimers meds and had him on antibiotics, his memory fog cleared and his glorious state of health began to return. I shudder to think how many other people are suffering the same ill fate.

Back to this present doctor doubting the positivity of my now fourth positive blood test confirming Lyme. As I sat there looking at his fancy desk, fancy watch, fancy computer with all the bells and whistles, burgeoning staff, and pricey address, I remembered reading online to be wary of misdiagnosis and the rabbit hole it leads you down, all to the tune of hundreds of thousands of dollars for some people.

What should I think if he didn't believe this positive Lyme test from his own lab?

Ok, so I took the bait, and I asked, "Hmmm, so what do you think I have if I don't have Lyme?"

His reply, said with a very serious face, was "I don't know, but we can start running some tests to find out."

I silently nodded my head while my jammed thoughts were screaming, *"Really!"*

Luckily, I had done enough research on the Internet to know this was out there. Some doctors were actually doing this! It was my luck to be there with this one. *What should I think if he didn't believe this positive Lyme test from his own lab?* What tests *would* he believe from his own lab as he tried to reassign my illness to something more professionally profitable and less challenging to his license?

I just nodded my head as he spoke. Lyme had taken away my ability to have any spontaneous meaningful conversations. The thoughts were there and coming fast, but they would jam up in my head in a confusing mess, all pressing to find a way out in verbal language, but my mind had lost the switch to translate thoughts into words. My head was screaming thoughts and words that only circled round and round with no way out.

Finally, I stammered, "May I have a copy of this report from your labs, please?" Oh, yes, he was thrilled that I seemed to be listening compliantly to him—no rebuttal, just zombie compliancy, as Lyme can make you behave. He proudly worked his fancy computer, printed out my positive Lyme report right there on the spot, and handed it to me over the large expansive desk, certain I would seek more testing along with his sage counsel.

Wordlessly, I took the printed report he handed me, I stood up, I gathered my belongings, I turned around, and I walked directly out of his office. Talk about fraud. I'm sure the insurance company paid his padded bill. I never saw him again.

I had also called around to all the local LLMD naturopaths I could locate. They wanted payments of $800 to $1,000 up front just to walk in the door. Then they could start "testing" procedures, which would incur more costs. I had no money for that, only insurance, which these naturopaths and many doctors refused to take in association with Lyme related cases.

In addition, once these doctors knew that I *had* insurance, they refused to see me—even when I said I would pay out of my own pocket! I begged, pleaded, and cried, and they still refused to see me because they knew I *had* insurance! Some of the administrative staff in these offices were incredibly mean. I could not believe what was happening.

A quick online search will reveal much political in-fighting between the two camps of IDSA and LLMD. I again urge anyone trying to recover from Lyme disease and co-infections to stay out of the political wrangling which abounds until your health has returned to full volume. Be aware of all the facts but do not jump in the ring until you are well enough.

Again and again, defeated. The need for me to surrender arose. Listening more closely to the word of God, I just knew there had to be a solution some way, somehow.

UNLOCKING THE SECRETS ABOUT LYME

THE ANSWER POSSIBLY lies somewhere in the middle between pharmaceuticals and Mother Nature's herbals. There is a key element to comprehending Lyme's sneaky protective behavior that is missing from medical understanding. This missing link is not being addressed by the doctors or their medical treatments.

I discovered this missing link, along with many other beneficial breakthroughs, and designed a protocol for myself which I still use today.

After being diagnosed with Lyme and engaged in a five-year struggle working to cure myself of the devastating, sneaky, crafty, clever Lyme spirochetes and their co-infection friends, I found myself recovered with great success. I decided to help as many other people suffering from the same terrible situation as I could.

Living with the Lyme spirochete element penetrating bones, organs, soft tissue, and brain requires one to create a healing strategy that works for the long haul.

Everyone asks what did I do to recover my health from Lyme and co-infections? It seems so prevalent these days. Either someone has Lyme, has had Lyme, or knows someone with Lyme.

Before I answer this question, I take a deep breath in and exhale. Then I try to explain the process and what I had to go through to examine everything in my life pertaining to my health and well being and change everything about my lifestyle and nutrition that did not align with true health and well being as we understand it to be today.

It took years to review my daily habits, body, mind, and soul to decide what needed to change or shift. This vibrational realignment went deeper and deeper into every aspect of my life including nutrition, work, environment, friends and associates, leisure, and spiritual pursuits.

I still do this work with myself today.

SELF-RESPONSE-ABILITY

YOU DESERVE ONLY the best. Incorporating progressive, permanent lifestyle adjustment tools requires that we recommit every day to our focused goal of complete and total wellness. The prerequisite for this goal is a can-do attitude. You fall down; you stand back up. Brush yourself off and move forward. Everyone has strife and struggles throughout life. It is not what has happened to you that counts. It is how you *react* to it that matters. Choose to be a Victor! You Can Do This!

My mom used to tease me when I was growing up by saying, "Sue, the first hundred years are the hardest!" When times were really bad I would remember this saying and could at least give a little chuckle at this truth. Love and nurture yourself back to health. This too shall pass.

Questions to ask your heart and soul in times of reflection:

Do you really *want* to recover your health?

Do you give yourself *permission* to heal?

Many think this would be an automatic and obvious, resounding, unanimous *YES*! But for some, surprisingly, it is not.

For me it was always *YES*! I prefer to be a high-functioning, interesting, curious, positive, action oriented and active individual, instead of a sickly hermit, complaining and looking for enablers to trample me with stress and anxiety.

Wellness is my choice and my choice alone.

But the trouble was figuring out how to get from here to there. I relied on this quote often to carry me when I could no longer see the light:

> *Keep your face to the sunshine, and you will not*
> *see the shadows.*

—Helen Keller

Philosophical teachings, poetry, and wise psalms were all reminders that kept me moving forward. They kept me striving for answers even when those around me were saying I would never recover and the road ahead seemed dark and alone.

Here are some of the strategies I focused on:

You cannot build a sturdy house on a weak foundation.

Sort through survival issues and sort out family and cultural issues.

Clear out the clutter of outgrown habits.

If you wear out your body, where will you live?

By projecting issues back onto others and blaming others, this behavior then takes the focus off us. "Blame takes the focus off you!"

Passive-aggressive behavior can be quite manipulating and subtle.

One finger pointing out, three fingers pointing back: remember the importance of self-care efforts.

No blaming anyone else: it is up to me.

There is no magic pill: it is up to me.

Nor was there an option of surgery that would remedy the pain: it was up to me.

Sometimes certain people do not want us to recover. Our disability and dependency on them provides a connection for them.

Over and over again: *self-response-ability*

Really, truly, this is it! This is not a dress rehearsal! You're sitting on 'it,' sleeping in 'it.' When 'it' runs perfectly, quietly, like a well-oiled machine, we can carry on with all tasks and endeavors of everyday life without even a second thought. We often take 'it' for granted.

With the absence of our sparkling health we come to appreciate and understand that the quality of our longevity requires real and focused care. By employing specific guidelines for making healthier and better informed choices we improve the quality of our happy long life.

Naturally, the process of aging creates damage which impacts long-term efforts toward optimum health. We need to work on it everyday without judgment. If you miss-step here and there do not worry, just pick up where you left off and keep moving forward.

By allowing oneself to get out of balance our weakened state allows our defenses to flair. Maintaining an awareness of these undesirable behaviors will help to keep our inner balance and keep the focus moving forward to a place of purpose and intention. In my work as a licensed massage therapist I was able to recognize there are times when people actually do not want to recover. Yes, this thought is very disturbing. Yet it is true that some people seem to perceive derived benefits from their ill status. There is a payoff for them being chronically sick. I was very sure to double-check myself over this issue by identifying any deflecting behaviors which could sabotage my recovery.

TURN OFF, TIME OUT, TUNE IN—MEMORY LOSS

MEMORY LOSS AND the horror of our minds just shutting off,will challenge even the strongest of us. This is what I refer to as the austerity phase. In part it is an emptying out of thoughts and issues that are no longer necessary because we have outgrown their usefulness. I found this gave me room for new thoughts of Peace. With this slowing down, you fully realize that much of the perceived control over our life is really out of our hands and has been for a very long time.

Flower Essences can be a great aid to relieve much of the hidden emotional cysts deep within our body. Dr. Edward Bach created 38 flower essence remedies in the Bach remedy system. All of them were discovered in the 1920s and 1930s by Dr Edward Bach who was a well-known bacteriologist, physician and pathologist. Each remedy is associated with a basic human emotion. Dr. Bach felt that there was a specific personality type for people with chronic diseases such as Lyme. According to him, we tend to be martyrs, rescuers, caretakers, scattered, Type-A perfectionists who excel at people pleasing. They can also relate to suffering from the oldest child syndrome, martyring as a method of peacekeeping as well as having experienced one or more trauma of some kind. For example, in my case, one of my past traumas invoked survivors guilt for much of my life after our family home exploded and burned down claiming the lives of my father and sister.

The bottom line: We have too much energy going out and not enough coming in! Lyme forces us to address this deficiency head-on.

The loss of language and reasoning is extremely disconcerting, and I am hard-pressed to find a positive aspect to this situation. Only that we can let go of the bad thoughts along with the good. Then replace the bad thoughts with new good and positive thoughts. One must have patience and compassion for oneself until these symptoms abate.

When memory loss started to happen for me and continued to worsen, the resulting ramification was an increasingly limited independence for living day to day. Many of those who suffer severely with Lyme are holed up in someone's basement, or spare room, just so they can rest. These people are absolutely unable to work or take care of themselves at all. For several years I was one of these people living by the grace of other kind friends and family.

Life is cooperation. Its is community. It is all beings getting along. When one is so desperately ill, there is no room, or energy, for arguments, stress, grudges, or jealousies. Peace, quiet, and calm are what one needs to strive for in a daily living environment. Yet, within Lyme there is a rage element that distorts all boundaries of perceived offenses.

Losing my ability to effectively communicate issues with the same balanced intensity I had cultivated before Lyme, left me terribly frightened for years. Using heavy-metal detox programs was a recovery tool for rebounding from this dreadful symptom, as were the use of grounding tools, which still play an important role in my maintaining a non–Lyme-friendly inner terrain. Nutritionally I increased healthy fats such as coconut oil for brain support.

NOW YOU SEE IT, NOW YOU DON'T—HEAVY METALS

HEAVY METAL CONTAMINATION and neurological Lyme can have you existing within parallel realities through experiencing hallucinations. Hallucinations can appear and seem as real as anything before us. These surfaced for me with devastating effects approximately one and a half years into Lyme and co-infections.

What do you do when you think you have seen something and another person knows for a fact it was not there? This happened to me.

As the disability caused bedridden hours to grow from days into weeks and then weeks into months and then years, I would constantly try to rally and get back into my daily routine. One beautiful and peaceful fall day I decided to get tough with myself and motivate!

Yes, that was it! I convinced myself I just needed some tough love!

> *Get out of that bed, Suzen, and do something positive for yourself today! Get back out into the world! It's all waiting for you! You just have to go and get it! Now quit playing around and get out of bed, shower, dress, eat, and get going!*

And so went my self-talk …

Deciding this jumpstart was just what I needed to force myself back into wellness, I embarked upon a day long expedition to New York City to attend my favorite wellness industry convention at the Jacob Javits Center. Unfortunately, however, this activity was to bring about a symptom that terrified me to the bone.

Let me explain.

After a pleasant mid-morning car ride into the city listening to my *Language of God* tapes by Gregg Braden, I parked my car a few blocks away from the convention center. As I stood next to my car waiting for the attendant to return from parking the prior client's car, I made a mental note of my surroundings. There was a woman sitting in a chair inside a small neat office. Scanning beyond the door I noticed a small office window with a sign hanging below listing parking fees. Just outside this office and a few feet in front of me was a sandwich-board sign, approximately four feet high and four feet wide, listing the parking prices.

Hearing the attendant's approaching footsteps behind me, I turned to greet him and turn over my keys. In the process I made a second mental note of this large sandwich-board sign located between the office and my car. I told the attendant I would return in a few hours. He was kind and courteous as he took my keys, hopped into my car, and drove off into the nether regions of the parking garage.

After a leisurely two-hour visit throughout the display hall at the convention center, I was ready to start heading home. It was a gentle mid-afternoon stroll back to the garage where I handed the same attendant my ticket to retrieve my car.

Again I stood outside the office taking in my surroundings. The lady who had earlier been sitting in the office was now gone, the chair vacant, the office empty. Soon the attendant returned with my car. He hopped out, handed me my keys, and said the fee would be twenty dollars.

Immediately my mind switched to a state of fear about this interaction. I lost the ability to comprehend what a fair price would be and I did not remember how to complete this transaction. I stood frozen as my mind again sent swirling thoughts round and round in circles within my mind, unable to put those thoughts into words. I felt the panic and paranoia start to escalate within this growing confusion of anxiety.

The attendant stood patiently waiting for me to pay him. I was stunned. All of a sudden my mind was convincing me something was wrong. I was being ripped off! My mind was convincing me that I was in danger. Again the attendant patiently said, "Twenty dollars, please, ma'am."

My mind started to splinter off with my next inquiry to the attendant, "Where is the sign that was here with the prices I saw earlier?" as I waved my hand in the empty space just outside the office. With a quizzical tilt of his head he replied, "What sign? There was no sign, ma'am."

A small fear gripped my senses as a little voice inside began questioning my own judgment. I brushed it away and continued, "There was a big sign here, right here—a sandwich-board sign with all the prices … I know I saw it … Where is it?" Now my mind is telling me I'm being tricked, fooled, there really was a sign and he hid it while I was gone!!!! I'm torn between believing and not believing my own eyes.

Becoming a bit frustrated, the attendant again explained there was never any such sign. He insisted that I walk to the top of the driveway entrance with him to see the enormous sign with prices posted high up right at the entrance wall—no one could miss it. No, that was not the sign I was talking about.

I thanked him for showing me this sign but said this was not what I was thinking of. We walked back down to my car, and I kept describing this sandwich-board sign.

As we approached the car the attendant carefully and directly looked me straight in the eye and said, "Ma'am, there was no sign. I would not lie to you. I am a God-fearing man, and I saw that you were listening to *The Language of God*. I am not lying to you. There was no sign." Half of me knew he was telling me the truth. The other half believed he was lying and, in my Lyme delusion, I would prove it!

For one final confirmation that I did in fact know what I was talking about, I whirled around to point my finger at the office window where I remembered having seen the other price sign earlier as well.

I blinked my eyes as I stopped mid-sentence. What I thought I had seen was not there! Oh no...my God..where was the window and sign?

Instead of seeing an office window and pricing sign hanging below, I saw a smoothly painted, rich brown, solid cinderblock wall. No window. No sign. Just a plain, clean, perfectly painted wall staring me back in the face.

Stunned and embarrassed, I fearfully looked into his eyes, swallowed, and quietly whispered pleadingly for confirmation. Was he sure? I really needed him to be sure there were no signs. I was beginning to realize something was seriously wrong with me.

Great sadness entered his eyes as he realized my truly confused state. He gently said, "I know, there was no sign" and with a silent confirmation from his kind eyes, he conveyed that yes, indeed, there was something terribly wrong with me.

I gasped. I paid him. And as he helped me get into my car, I realized that there could not have been a sandwich-board sign where I thought I had seen one. There was not enough room in the garage entry for both a car and a sign. The car would have run the sign over. I drove up the ramp and out into the city streets. I was facing a two-hour drive home and did not know if I would make it safely.

Thankfully it was a beautiful day, and the mid-afternoon traffic was light. I do not even remember the trip home. Once there I undressed and found my first bulls-eye type rash. It was approximately eight inches in diameter located on my lateral left mid-back beneath my shoulder blade. Over the years several types of rashes would come and go in different areas of my body but this was the first sign of a bulls-eye rash since being bitten 1.5 years earlier. I put on my pajamas and went right to bed, stunned with this newest development. I cried and was ready to surrender to this disease, not because Lyme had won but rather because I had discovered that it was bigger than me, bigger than the doctors, and bigger than the medical community—bigger than anyone realized. My fear was that maybe there really was no answer, maybe there was no cure. It was many years before I would fully recover.

Unless you have or have had Lyme, you just cannot comprehend the enormity of this disease and the frightening fear that wrecks your body daily, only varying by one degree or another.

I eventually learned to relax myself with inspired meditation music and self-created visualizations of a higher order. I tried to spend time being grateful within this "letting go" austerity phase. I tried to focus on not so much pushing out, but rather a focus to refine the art of going within and breathing into deeper layers.

Inflammation was rampant within my body and brain causing much trouble. Working to soothe this tissue inflammation is a major step in recovering my ability for clarity and communication. What role does diet and nutrition play? Histamine triggers can be found with food sensitivities to processed foods, sugar, high fructose corn syrup, nightshades, gluten including holy wafers, lipstick, canned soups, GMO wheat, corn, soy, antibiotic pumped dairy and meat, and hidden toxic ingredients found in body care and cleaning products. These acid-forming substances are major contributing factors to chronic inflammation. Keeping a food and lifestyle journal helped me identify and discover what habits needed to be eliminated in order to enhance my wellness protocol.

We have already discussed the impact negative relationships have on our health. Keeping this daily journal kept track of where I was emotionally stuck so I could allow more healing to take place around these sensitive issues.

I also cultivated an intentional, calming, daily mindset on my healing journey relating to my strategic solutions for tick-free zones. These tools include tick keys, lavender oil, diatomaceous earth, cedar wood chip borders around the lawn, safe dressing by tucking clothes in socks and boots and wearing hats. With these safety issues covered I could relax and enjoy my days.

I focused on physical endurance even if it meant only walking outside to the end of the walk and back due to shear exhaustion. Self-discipline required I at least try once a day.

Who is running the show, you or the spirochetes? Keep a journal answering these questions and others that you can think of:

- What are the effects on your mind and personality?
- How does it affect rages, depression, anxiety, joy, and happiness?
- What about scars on the brain? Are they related to Alzheimer's, type-3 diabetes, or high iron content?
- What about neurological Lyme visual impairment?
- Is your thought process in vibrational alignment with your congruent integrity?
- What are your dream goals?
- What self-care tools do you engage to manage, limit, and monitor flare-ups?
- What does increased oxygen accomplish for you?
- Are you regularly grounded?
- What is the physical damage left behind from Lyme and how do you intend to remedy it?
- What is your upgraded level of awareness, action, and purpose?
- What are your self-empowerment techniques?
- What does it mean to "stand in your truth"?
- How do you support immune enhancement and what is a herxing strategy for recovery?
- How do you find time to attend local Lyme support groups?
- What is your first step in beginning the healing journey?
- What are your chess game strategy and surrender maneuvers ?
- What are the orders of healing strategy? What are first, second, and third?
- Regarding economics, how will you prioritize spending?

- What are boutique healing tools, therapies and routines—bells and whistles, for later in the recovery?
- Are homeopathic and herbal remedies effective and working for you at full capacity?
- Have you eliminated fluoride from toothpaste, water, tea which have been watered with fluoride-laced water, white tea bags, and the like?
- What is causing inflammatory pain flare-ups—viruses, bacteria, or repetitive stress?
- What is the life cycle pattern of spirochetes in your body?
- What foods are you eating that feed spirochetes?
- What starves spirochetes?
- What supports your immune system?
- Which, if any, co-infection do you have?
- Have you found that probiotics change your brain activity or emotional responses?
- Are you using a tongue scraper to stimulate the gag reflex? This reconnects the gut-brain connection by stimulating the vagus nerve.

THE IMPORTANCE OF UNIVERSAL ORDER

THE MOST COMMONLY shared health component of those who heal is to cultivate their best mindset.

Be flexible and strong like young bamboo.

Start doing the next thing in front of you, and go from there.

Regarding old injuries, work your way back toward the beginning of root causes.

Focus and be disciplined. For extraordinary focus, dial in on a few things that bring greatest value. As a result, you will work less and live more.

Enjoy the journey along the way. The cause of death is life itself.

Start small, use steady increments, and consistently build over time. All health in life is a process of continuous improvements. Solving a problem inch by inch proves everything is manageable; but done yard by yard, everything proves to hard and discouraging with enormity.

One hundred percent commitment and focus adhering to an increasingly clean and balanced lifestyle is required for at least three months in the beginning before you may see marked improvement. Each day I tried to discover and implement something beneficial. There was always a forward and backward movement during the healing journey.

Soon enough you will reach the halfway point in your recovery where the first half seemed so slow, like it would never happen. Once you reach the halfway point you will feel an acceleration of your wellness recovery journey. Your joy will start to return, your happiness will rebound, and your energy will become bountiful and vibrant!

There will be some back and forth along the way but do not be discouraged. Just keep moving forward with a positive attitude.

By the end of the final phase of recovery and rebuilding vitality, you will bounce and shine with a smile that makes others wonder what your special secret to happiness is.

Once my health was back on steady ground, I developed a maintenance program of an 80/20 strategy: 80 percent of your results come from 20 percent of your activities. Keep your top 20 percent good habits and discontinue 80 percent of your bad habits, and watch your health go up and disease go down.

The key is to find your unique area of vibrational support for your own body. Explore what other people are doing for their best practices. Then, incorporate those behaviors and see if they improve your results. Not everything will work for everyone.

Compile a list from one to ten of the good things you do. Next, make a list from one to ten of your worst habits. Now refer to this list often and be sure to focus on eliminating the negative habits and increase the beneficial habits.

Zero-based thinking has a goal of restructuring and reinvesting in activities based on asking yourself the following question:

If I knew what I know now, would I do those activities again?

Do those activities increase or decrease your stress, pain, or anxiety?

As you begin to heal with these tools, your body will teach you how to more accurately adjust your lifestyle.

Evaluate relationships both personal and professional in the same way. How fast can you move away from the toxic, stressful elements and how quickly and congruently can you change to enforce new, healthy habits?

How can you anchor in new habits and lifestyle?

Which routines and lifestyle activities either support or deplete your body's efficiency in handling the Lyme and co-infection toxic overload.

How can you dramatically increase efficient and supportive elements in your life?

1) Clarify your goals and design action steps. Consistently work to support an ideal lifestyle. What does that look like for you? What are the steps you must take to reach that goal?

2) Simplify your life consistently as much as possible in every area. Make a list of all activities that support your goal, and do those things.

3) Make a list of all the harmful activities, and eliminate those activities as soon as possible.

4) Leverage access to other peoples resources and skills. Delegate, outsource, or eliminate as much as you can. Be flexible, open, and optimistic. Ask for help.

5) Accelerate your healing by focusing on a 100 percent lifestyle improvement list. Think things through before you begin activities. Do the most important items first and accept that you have limits. Love yourself just where you are. Do not be afraid to say NO.

6) Gently multiply those activities and habits that support and create the most healthy, successful outcomes in how you want to feel. Nourish the roots of healthy activities. Invest in yourself and your recovery. Remember, each new piece of information can accelerate your recovery. You are worth it.

7) Maximize the latest technologies and the highest quality products. Only deal with the best of the best. The highest-quality

resources will ensure the purest quality and the highest vibration for the most powerful healing protocol.

8) Leverage your time and efforts through research and incorporation of new tools that appear safe and beneficial. Ask questions, and design the best action blueprint for your personal recovery.

9) Review these items frequently and make adjustments where necessary for building support protocols.

Work this plan for three months and then review, revise, and repeat for the next three months. Concentrate on your top 20 percent activities each time and look for 80 percent results.

When you become comfortable with each new lifestyle tool, aim for 100 percent incorporation. This is why it is important to design a slower, steadier pace. It is not about how fast you recover. It is about the permanent positive results of the healing protocol.

Become a synthesizer of information from many sources. Constantly distill and discern the best techniques that empower you to generate positive forward momentum on your life's joyous journey.

As healing acceleration continues, you will be able to move forward evermore quickly and efficiently through relapses. These relapses will in turn themselves decrease with time and patience as you refine your personal protocol preferences.

If you really want to have a successful, healthy recovery from Lyme disease and co-infections, find out what really works and do that!

Resolutely work at it everyday, allowing grace to enter and soften those harsh relapses that command you to redouble your efforts, again, starting with baby steps.

Throw your whole heart and soul into it, and *never give up*!

SELF-EMPOWERED HEALTH THROUGH CLARITY AND DISCERNMENT

Q. Will I ever be cured?

A. Only you will determine that outcome.

Q. How will I know if I am over Lyme disease and co-infections?

A. Your body will tell you with increased energy and decreased pain.

AWAKENING UPON AWAKENING will guide you to your next layer of healing. When you are ready to transform your health, your wealth, and your vitality through the stepping-up of lifestyle and nutrition and applying modifications by accepting self-response-ability, you are ready for this journey.

At the end of the day, you need to believe in your own ability to take control of your life and health. We can walk beside you, guide you, and cheer you on, but at the end of the day you alone can claim the prize of the power to heal from within.

A WORKABLE STRATEGY FOR RECOVERING YOUR HEALTH

A SUCCESSFUL LIFE is living your life with full joy and happiness based in gratitude and love. Sparkling health allows us to connect with this joy and happiness. Depletion, malabsorption and toxicity all lead to poor health and a disconnect from our true desires. Choose your desired path with focused intent.

> Pay now or pay later. Pay the farmer
> or pay the doctor.

The blood should be clean. Think of it as garden soil and cells as plants. Focus on clearing your organ filtration pathways, liver and gallbladder, to help form the purest access to elements that properly nourish cells allowing them to more fully absorb nutrients to support cellular metabolic function.

The lymph system should be addressed thoroughly as well. Lymph brings out the garbage from deep within our body and brain. When our lymph fluid is dirty and thick, we become constipated or perhaps our kidneys are not filtering properly, we are headed down a toxic path.

Journal progress questions:

What healing tools are working for you?

What is your definition of success?

What does a successful recovery look like and feel like for you?

What internal messages are you getting that you are ignoring?

How are you maintaining a victim or a Victor archetype?

These are all important questions for you to contemplate. Empower yourself by letting go of the guilt and resentment which keeps you from aligning with your focused desires. Procrastination is suicide on the installment plan. Complacency is death. If there is a hill to climb, waiting will not make it go away or make it any smaller. Learn to take responsibility for your feelings and use them to connect with spiritual love. Create your new reality and align with that vision. Do it now!

Do not let yourself be overcome by bad habits; instead, overcome them by forming good habits. Take care of what you have regarding your beautiful health.

When you start gaining what you positively believe you deserve, you start to live your life's purpose. Your health is your wealth. If enough damage has occurred within the body, it could eventually reach a level where no amount of money or effort can help you regain your optimum health.

Form the God habit! In his book 'Daylight Diet,' Paul Nison has a powerful message regarding the health laws written in the Bible. I never knew there were instructions from our Creator written in the Holy Bible. Paul has generously published many You Tube videos which were my lifeline for getting clear on these Divinely inspired health laws.

Some of these changes were eating the most calories during the daylight hours. Eating late at night was working against me and feeding the Lyme which grew at night. I stopped processed foods and started consuming organic raw foods as much as possible. I found it was not possible to be completely raw during the winter months up here in New England. I would say 80% was raw salads and fresh juices with 20% following a loosely fitted blood type diet. My inner light started to shine again.

One of my favorite therapists who helped me overcome and manage my PTSD when it first reared its ugly head, had two great items in her office which influenced me greatly. One was a poster which stated '*If you wear out your body, where will you live?*' So true when you really think about the consequences of one's actions. The other was '<u>Are You My Mother?</u>' by Dr. Seuss.

These two sayings reminded me that much of my people-pleasing behaviors, rooted in survivors guilt, overrode my gut instinct for self-care. Contemplating these stark concepts helped me learn to stop fighting myself and surrendering more and more to increasing self-care — social consequences be dammed! It had to be done or I would be done!

Practice daily clean living in all areas of life, including nutrition, work, home, and spiritual life. Each area of these life categories needs continual balancing to maintain continued wellness. Self-love which leads to quality self-care is the key to this breakthrough. Therefore, rescuing and care-taking of others is not loving ourselves if our needs are not met first, and leading to further self-depletion.

We must realize that self-care is not selfish. People may get really mad at you because they have grown accustomed to being served in such a way. The best loving people will stay in your life and support your new found self-care and self-love. The self-serving people who drain your energy will eventually fall away. Eat the foods that nourish you and tell the people you love that you Love them.

PREVENTION IS THE BEST CURE

THE PINEAL GLANDULAR portal connects our lower consciousness to our higher consciousness. When we ingest fluoride from our public water supply, toothpaste, dental procedures, pharmaceuticals, white tea bags, and more, our pineal gland becomes calcified. Thereby, we are then unable to access our higher consciousness. This is just one example of how environmental toxins enter our body and interfere with the body's ability to keep its inner terrain pristine and working perfectly.

All environmental toxins count, including mercury and other heavy metals, flame retardant fumes, out-gassing from new materials, BPA plastic bottles, EMFs, dirty electricity, chem-trails, Fukushima fallout, and, sadly, so much more.

Lyme has a tendency to cause *extreme* environmental sensitivity for many individuals. This most challenging condition can be managed with time and patience. Following Lyme I found that I was completely unable to handle odors from chemicals, mold, cigarette smoke, etc. Before Lyme I could roll in Poison Ivy with no bad affects. Now all I have to do is look at it and I get it! Life is challenging and painful for sufferers. Others perhaps will lack compassion and a willingness to assist during episodes of relapse. You must be strong within and not allow them to shake your confidence or instill doubt. If they are not part of the solution they are part of the problem. You are on your personal healing journey. Keep your focus on the fact that you will recover.

We have seen an increase in the population of ticks, Lyme disease, and co-infections. I wonder if this is partly due to the increase in EMF towers and dirty electricity in general. Cell phones and Wi-fi agitate our body. So too, they agitate the spirochetes. Restless, the spirochete hide and replicate.

Five-ninth graders carried out a science fair experiment showing how Wi-fi and cell phone radiation is harmful to living organisms. The girls had already noticed that if they slept with their cell phones next to their head, they had trouble concentrating in school the next day.

Their experiment involved using some watercress seeds. They put half in a room with no Wi-fi coming in, and the other half in a room next to two Wi-fi routers. The watercress in the Wi-fi-free room grew nicely, but the watercress next to the Wi-fi routers did not grow, and most died.

On holiday my children came to visit armed with laptop movie capabilities to stave off boredom here in the country. Each of them now live in an upbeat metropolitan area. They do not necessarily enjoy "unplugging" while visiting Mom's out-of-service area. They are tight-knit and dedicated to one another's welfare. When the hustle-and-bustle holidays roll around, relaxing time together is precious.

While visiting, they were trying for quite a while to get the Wi-fi connection going and not having much luck. I produced the modem security code to assist. Bummer—still not working Ma! The Wi-fi modem box sits on my desk. I did a bit of fiddling around with no results. Okay, now they were getting a wee bit frustrated!

Grounding is a technique I adopted to heal body aches and pains from Lyme. Grounding facilitates our direct physical connection to the earth. Standing in bare feet on the earth, but not on asphalt, cement or rubber, this raw connection to the earth aligns our inner terrain negative ions.

Now remembering I habitually unplug the Wi-fi connection to reduce my exposure to EMFs, I quickly reattach the Wi-fi connection cord, and bravo! Power! And now again I hear it from the relieved but disgruntled peanut gallery: "Mom! Why do you do that! Besides, it's no use—there are EMFs all over these days, so you're not doing anything when you do that, except make it harder to get movies!"

EMFs, otherwise known as electromagnetic fields, emit pulses into the airwaves so we can have cell phone service, Wi-fi service, drive-by meter reading and the like. These frequencies agitate our bodies and seem to be turning up everywhere. Point taken, yes, sadly I do comprehend we are now in a world where it is virtually impossible to avoid EMFs, smart meters, dirty electricity, and the like. Meters have shown that even if a light is turned off, it is still drawing and emitting EMFs. To my way of thinking, that is all the more reason to unplug all electronics which would disturb my sleep and ground whenever I can.

Back to the Internet connection, it was up and working but not running well. Daughter One was growing testy as she tried to FaceTime with her friend at the Hong Kong tailors as there were some very important details she needed to review! Eventually, she gave up.

Still having no luck with the movie connection, after trying for almost another hour, we settled on ordering a movie on-demand. Then, after all that fussing, they all promptly fell asleep not fifteen minutes into the purchased movie!

By morning we discovered the true awesome power of using tinfoil as an EMF deterrent when I remembered that not only did I *unplug* the Wi-fi modem on the desk when not in use, but I also *covered* the unit completely with tinfoil when it was actually plugged in and in use. I was not sure but I had a hunch this might truly cancel out EMF output exposure. Now we saw that it actually did work! And I sure did get another earful from the kids, because as soon as I removed the tinfoil from the Wi-fi modem, everything was back up and running. FaceTime was up and working and movies were available for the taking.

True to my form, as soon as they left, I unplugged the Wi-fi modem and replaced the tinfoil covering the unit, happy with the knowledge that my techniques really do work!

WHAT THE HEALING PATH LOOKS LIKE

HEALING IS DIFFERENT from curing. Curing is what our current medical society provides for us as an answer for our expressed desire to live our life disease free. They employ medications along with medical treatments and interventions in their attempts to obtain our desired goal. We turn our money and our will over to their trusted care. For some portion of our population this is sufficient and good.

But for others, they more hear the chant 'you are a master piece because you are a piece of the master'. Healing for them is paramount. Healing is an internal process which balances our body, mind and souls spiritual energy in our quest for wholeness. Effective healing tools are essential when the negative influences of illness, loss, or life challenges encompass our life.

The ultimate benefit of recovery from Lyme is a personal Quantum energetic recalibration through awakening upon awakening to our inner truths. If we are sincerely thorough in our healing efforts, it has the potential to actually propel us faster along our spiritual alignment and ascension journey.

The five stages of recovery from Lyme disease and co-infections for me were:

1) reduction of spirochete population and toxic load
2) fibromyalgia
3) chronic fatigue
4) recovery and increasing individual vitality
5) deeper connection to my *soul's purpose thru balanced body, mind, spirit*

This new found deeper self-awareness allows spontaneity which allows miraculous healing. This is accomplished through Love.

An explanation of phase conjugation is that where bacterial rods with electrical impulses cross over one another, they absorb each others qualities and coding in a spiral movement, which is then creating and created around the resulting core gravity. The core essence that is created by this intermingling and compression of phase conjugation is LOVE.

Furthermore, healing vibrations are beautifully confirmed in Emoto's Hidden Messages In Water. Therefore again, we look at Lyme as a chess opponent whereby we dismantle forces through a love strategy, not nuclear war of antibiotics.

Dealing with grief after the loss of our once high-functioning life, can leave us feeling extra vulnerable. Focus as much as possible on self-care to help fortify the self against this painful tide.

The five stages of grief are

1) denial
2) anger
3) bartering
4) acceptance
5) assimilation

Buddha reminds us nothing is permanent. On good days we want happiness to stay always, but this cannot be. For just as happiness will flee, so too will sadness flee after it has sat a while in our world.

Remember to give yourself permission to be just who you are. It is the right time to stand in your truth without the need for others approval. Learn to say NO.

Impermanence is the word of the day in this ebb and flow.

Do not let other people rent space in your mind.

Follow the word of God.

Keep positive in thought.

Recognize that when we choose the behavior, we choose the consequences.

Finding the good in people bolsters spiritual compassion. Love is the grand prize in life. It is also the way to tap into the gift in Lyme disease.

Our different life experiences color each individuals filter, as if a fog on a mirror, through which life is viewed. The unawakened unaware unexamined unconscious soul reacts from a place of raw emotion. The evolved and purposefully awakened soul will pause a moment to reflect and come from a more Universal source.

When you need a rest from all the healing work you are doing within yourself, take time to rest quietly. When it does come time to make plans to be near people, be with those who are easy to be with. Avoid energy vampires who drain you. Visit with ones who laugh, smile, and can have easy breezy conversations which restore self radiance in light.

Louise Hay's book *You Can Heal Your Life* has been a staple for my active massage practice, and now it serves to support my navigation of Lyme's effect on my body. The where and why of all I was feeling. Being that Lyme proliferates in an internal systemic acidic environment, Louise's book helps to trace past-emotional experiences that have weakened us through physical manifestation of these issues into our body.

We can begin to ask questions in relation to these challenges and ask how to overcome them with clearer emotional fortitude. It becomes an individualized recipe when adding, integrating, and distilling combined therapeutic modalities.

Astrology can add clarity when we study the human body parts that have been assigned to astrological signs and relate them to human nature.

Astrological Anatomy: Body Rulership

Aries	Head
Taurus	Throat
Gemini	Arms
Cancer	Hands
Leo	Heart
Virgo	Stomach
Libra	Kidneys
Scorpio	Pelvis
Sagittarius	Thighs
Capricorn	Knees/legs
Aquarius	Ankles
Pisces	Feet

Reading the body's pain signals will allow a deep view into our inner emotional terrain and correct the course of action. We strive for alignment with our true vibrational path by sensing and taking the path of least resistance. When we are out of alignment with sources deliverance for us, we experience fear and blockages.

Eastern healing modalities are provided in the nutrient chart listed below. It is a valuable map for when pain clues lead us to inquire what our bodies are trying to communicate.

For example, awakening between the hours of 3 a.m. and 5 a.m. happens within the Lung meridian timeframe, which represents grief in Chinese medicine. If we have recently lost a loved one, we may well find ourselves awakened during these hours as we process our emotional overload due to this loss.

Involving Quantum healing, disease does have a starting point as a ripple effect within the auric field originating from thought. We can become accustomed to this disturbance and believe that it is normal to adapt our lifestyle to work around this misalignment. If we ignore it for too long, we reach a tipping point where the pain of our dis-ease overwhelms us as it manifests into a misaligned physical form and disease. At that point we cannot always depend on medications alone to assist in our recovery. The answer to healing does not exist outside of itself. The answer lies within.

The Nutrient Cycle and Cycle of Tides

Arm Great Yin Lung	Metal	3 a.m. through 5 a.m.
Arm Bright Yang Colon	Metal	5 a.m. through 7 a.m.
Leg Bright Yang Stomach	Earth	7 a.m. through 9 a.m.
Leg Great Yin Spleen	Earth	9 a.m. through 11 a.m.
Arm Lesser Yin Heart	Fire	11 a.m. through 1 p.m.
Arm Great Yan Small Intestine	Fire	1 p.m. through 3 p.m.
Leg Great Yan Urinary Bladder	Water	3 p.m. through 5 p.m.
Leg Lesser Yin Kidney	Water	5 p.m. through 7 p.m.
Arm Absolute Yin Heart Envelope	Fire	7 p.m. through 9 p.m.
Arm Lesser Yang San Jiao	Fire	9 p.m. through 11 p.m.
Leg Lesser Yang Gall Bladder	Wood	11 p.m. through 1 a.m.
Leg Absolute Yin Liver	Wood	1 a.m. through 3 a.m.

Five Element Correspondences

Relative Phase	Yin Viscera	Yang Bowels	Sense Organ	Tissue	Color	Emotion	Season	Climate
Fire	Heart	Small intestine	Tongue	Blood vessels	Red	Over-excited joy	Summer	Heat
Earth	Spleen	Stomach	Mouth	Flesh	Yellow	Worry, excess thinking	Change of season	Damp
Metal	Lung	Colon	Nose	Skin, hair	Ash White	Sadness	Autumn	Dryness
Water	Kidney	Urinary bladder	Ear	Bones	Black	Fear	Winter	Cold
Wood	Liver	Gallbladder	Eye	Tendon	Green	Anger	Spring	Wind

Meridians are specific pathways throughout the body that enable chi to travel freely. Chi carries the electrical impulse that ignites our energy. It is also the emotional doorway to the soul. Maintaining unblocked energy flow through the meridians is important. This prevents the development of energy cysts, which can create problems over time.

Our body uses pain as a communication system to indicate a lack of homeostasis. Where there is pain, there is a problem.

As our pain levels increase, so too does the effect upon our nervous system. The longer and more intensely we suffer with this pain, the greater the damage and the harder it will be to repair. Checking to see if cells have good methylation capabilities regarding folic acid and B vitamins, will aid in repairing damaged nerves causing the neuropathy.

The 'Barking Dogs' pain scale rates the degree of discomfort from zero, which would be feeling well, to ten, registering extreme pain. The longer we endure the pain the more sensitive we become to triggers tapping into this pain pattern.

For example, if your body consistently registers a neuropathy pain pattern at nine, and you start a program to reduce that neuropathy pain pattern, it is important to realize it will take time for this sensitive triggered area to diminish response levels. It will take time for the nerve pathways to heal as the inflammation is contained and reduced. Until the healing is more complete, the slightest trigger can cause the nerve pain to register back up to nine or higher, even though you are progressing through your protocol.

We need to keep working on healing the damaged nerve pathways. B vitamins and folic acid are beneficial for nerve healing. Yellow and orange fruits and vegetables will aid in repair. Green vegetables will oxygenate and deodorize. Black foods are high in zinc and will rebuild kidneys and restore core energy.

A FEW FACTS ABOUT THE BODY

OUR BODIES ARE electric and water is the conduit. These electrical impulses run all throughout our body as well as on myelin sheaths designed for nerve communication speed. These impulses are the spark of life performing entwined duties such as stimulating our autonomic heartbeat.

Myofascial tissue is similar to a body stocking that surrounds every cell, every organ, and every muscle fiber in our body. You could form a hologram of the entire body from just a piece of this tissue. If you have ever looked closely at a piece of chicken and seen the whitish connective tissue, that is myofascial tissue. It holds everything in its place and optimally allows segments of the body to glide smoothly over one another.

Leafy green veggies and coconut water are fabulous for their electromagnetic enhancement properties. So I make every effort to incorporate these items in my primary food regime.

Structure Is Function, and Function Is Structure

In my healing work I find it helpful to provide a description of the anatomy and physiology for those who are healing. I stated earlier, our past physical and emotional traumas leave their mark upon and within us, following each traumatic event. Emotional events create energy cysts which can become embedded within soft tissue and remain there undetected causing vibrational issues for years on end. Physical trauma to soft tissue will leave compromised scar tissue, also causing problems. These injured areas receive restricted nourishment and become extremely acidic. Lyme will settle into these areas because they thrive in acidic low oxygenated areas.

Inactivities such as sleeping and excessive eating of sugar and processed foods, food sensitivities, and emotional trauma will all cause a fuzz to develop in between the myofascial tissue layers, thereby, causing the gliding action to freeze between these layers.

Restrictive scar tissue from physical trauma develops by the body forming a crisscross, fuzzy thatch-work of reinforcing, ill-fitting fibers which help to reinforce soft tissue, yet in doing so, restrict movement. In the event of soft tissue trauma the myofascial tissue, which acts like cling wrap, gets crinkled-up and pulls from all other parts of the body. This causes structural misalignment and further blockages. This can be remedied with cross-fiber tissue massage applied to the myofacial scar tissue.

Reducing these adhesions and facilitating easier flowing fiber movement pleasantly results in an increase of easy, pain-free movement. Pain, muscle aches and arthritic conditions are helped greatly by self-massage if you have the energy to do it. Pain arises in the soft tissue for various reasons and with this basic understanding you, or a caregiving loved one, can affect great relief.

Picture the soft tissue muscle bundle to be like a bunch of spaghetti strands all lined up together. Each individual muscle fiber is encased in their own myofascial tissue sleeve. Then another layer of myofascial tissue encases the entire muscle bundle group to form specific muscle groups such as the biceps, obliques or gastrocnemius. These muscles are attached to skeletal bone and facilitate movement through agonist/antagonist action, like a push/pull or gas/brake action.

There are two proprioceptor fibers associated with muscle and muscle/bone attachment sites which are responsible for adjusting muscle tension. They are the muscle spindle, which is a fiber within the muscle belly, and the Golgi-tendon organ located within the tendon. When either of these fibers are massaged with a cross-fiber technique, the result will be to improve the tone of the muscle.

Pain develops where the scar tissue impairs electrical impulses from passing through the meridians. This blockage causes depletion and undernourishment and therefore weaker body tissue as time goes on.

A charlie-horse cramp results when individual muscle fibers repeatedly splinter and break due to overuse and inadequate rest to complete the healing process. As muscles are used, fibers naturally break. When this happens, other healthy fibers rally around the splintered one and stiffen for support to prevent further damage. This protective stiffening impedes nourishing blood flow to the damaged area. If a damaged muscle is used before sufficient rest and repair has taken place, further damage will occur with the surrounding undernourished muscle fibers, which will then also start to break.

Now we have a cycle developing where, the next layer of muscle fibers surrounding these prior, damaged fibers, are recruited to rally around and stiffen for added structural support. Then next around those damaged fibers are more damaged fibers because of insufficient rest and repair. That is the Charlie-horse formation - layer upon layer upon layer of damaged scaring tissue.

Again this action, in turn, continues to cut off the blood flow that carries all the nutrients and oxygen necessary to rebuild body tissue. This pain syndrome is called pain-spasm-pain cycle.

Without proper rest and time for repair this pain-spasm-pain cycle continues, getting bigger and bigger at each turn. Muscular pain of this kind is one of the most excruciating feelings within the body. Magnesium will help restore soft tissue constitution, it will help you sleep and have proper bowel movements as well. Magnesium/Baking Soda/Sea Salt baths are a great way to absorb magnesium and detox toxins.

Our skeleton provides structure for our upright movement and walking-around capability. Muscles attach to skeletal bones and work in pairs to enable us to move. The pairing works by way of an agonist/antagonist method. In other words, one muscle relaxes while the opposite muscle tightens. And then the tight muscle relaxes while the relaxed muscle tightens for the reverse movement.

When there is an imbalance due to traumatic tissue disturbance the resulting myofascial tissue pulls and will affect this muscle-pairing dance. The body produces inflammation and pain to indicate a need for attention and rebalancing in these areas.

Viruses and bacteria cause inflammation in soft tissue, such as carpel tunnel. We can work with this buried pain to access greater health instead of having it block our pathway to greater health. To do this we focus on healing the area of soft tissue disturbance from trauma or we can address our energy cysts of fear or shame from emotional traumas which the resulting pain is covering up. Our acidic inner-terrain is the key to healing trauma trapped within.

Self massage for the pain-spasm-pain cycle is nicely accomplished with cross-fiber massage and is quite simple. To do this locate the muscle belly giving you trouble. Now locate the two distal sites of the muscle's attachment to bone. Returning to the belly of this muscle place your thumb pad first gently on this area. As you begin to apply deeper pressure, gently rub your thumb back and forth in a sideways motion to separate the muscle fibers.

The main focus of massage in general is to separate the fibers so nutrient rich blood will rush back into these areas and nourish the damaged tissue for rejuvenation. After this muscle belly is massaged we next address the tendons which attach the muscle to the bone. For this place thumb on the tendon and rub back and forth. This will stimulate the golgi tendon organ and facilitate muscle balance.

Another beneficial therapy for addressing structural muscle spasms and arthritic conditions from Lyme is chiropractic care. This therapy is an essential component of the healing journey in recovery from neurological Lyme and the terribly ugly, bone-gnawing soft-tissue pain experienced from *Bartonella*.

One of the most severe neurological pain patterns from neurological chronic Lyme is Trigeminal neuralgia (TN), also known as tic douloureux. It is considered to be among the most painful of conditions endured by mankind with nerve pain being so severe that many choose the option of suicide to get out from under this painful condition. But wait my friends there is a kinder, gentler way to assuage and heal here.

Trigeminal neuralgia is the result of the inflammation of this fifth cranial nerve through irritation. The TN supplies almost the entire face with sensation. The resulting pain arising in different areas of the face gives TN the distinction of being the most frequent of all neuralgias. Thankfully it can be remedied with application of ice packs, neti- pot, enemas and chiropractic care.

Correct alignment between soft tissue and bony structures supports and sets down correct energetic and neuronal pathways.

Acupuncture, acupressure and cranial sacral massage will aid in rebalancing the physical body too by addressing the cranial sacral fluids. These therapies combined with chiropractic care will really help move healing forward.

To spinal tap or not to spinal tap? When I first got sick I went to two top IDSA doctors before knowing about the controversy at that time surrounding Lyme disease and treatments. My first IDSA doctor referred me to my second IDSA doctor who was a prominent neurologist. After his evaluation of my condition and records, he advised against my having a spinal tap. I am very grateful for his guidance. He suggested it might introduce more problems for several reasons, all for the same conclusion - Lyme had me down for the count.

Massage is always lovely, relaxing and nourishing but I would reserve several types of massage for later in the healing journey or to not do at all.

My thought is to avoid Swedish massage in the beginning due to the high rate of blood and lymphatic movement, which is what Swedish massage is known for. This action would spread the spirochetes around the body faster and into places they may not have gone to until later stages of development, if at all. Add to this, a clogged lymphatic system and you just have a toxic soup mix. Use your judgment as to the phase you are in and if Swedish would be advantageous or not.

As it is taught today, one massage technique I avoid in general is lymphatic massage. This specific type of massage erroneously directs lymphatic fluid back towards the heart into the vena cava. This reintroduction of lymphatic waste back into the core of the circulatory system is contributing to an offensive and already high acidic state. Along with further taxing the Lyme heart and provoking Postural Orthostatic Tachycardia Syndrome (POTS), it completely ignores the fact that the brain also has its own lymphatic fluid system.

That is a big problem because as we discussed earlier, blood is the kitchen providing nourishment for cellular metabolism. Lymphatic fluid mucus is the sewage disposal fluid to clear out the debris from the cellular metabolism and toxic waste circulating around our body everyday.

So if we massage the lymphatic fluid back towards the heart, we are, therefore, mixing the sewage back into the blood as it is presently taught and utilized for lymphatic massage. We are basically dumping the sewage directly back into our blood stream. It makes no sense. This action also increases an acidic state of the blood causing further inflammation and continuing the biofilm potential for expansion.

Holistic Healing Is Accepting Full Responsibility for Our Own Role in Our Own Healing
—Suzen Chan

A very important component of healing is comprehending the concept of the harmonic resonance of hertz measurements, which is the light frequency something or someone is made up of in relation to that which is around itself. This transformative concept was explained beautifully, in part, by both Deepak Chopra and Gregg Braden regarding Quantum healing when taught to me decades ago.

Everything is vibration. If we were small enough we would fit right through these harmonically resonating gaps in the wall, the chair, literally everything. This all-is-one consciousness is derived from the total count volume of vibrational units of each Hz vibrational resonance.

For example a rose has 320 Hz, lavender has 118 Hz, myrrh has 105 Hz and our heart-love resonates with a span of 432 Hz and 528 Hz. All these tools are proven to create healing vibrations for the body, mind and spirit.

Flower Essence Therapy is a profound healing tool used to address embedded energy cysts which have resulted from past emotional traumas and are causing blockages. Once these energy cysts are released you are free from the spiritual chains and hungry ghosts of the past as well told in this story of two monks on their journey written here by Ahlhalau.

A senior monk and a junior monk were traveling together. At one point, they came to a river with a strong current. As the monks were preparing to cross the river, they saw a very young and beautiful woman also attempting to cross. The young woman asked if they could help her cross to the other side.

The two monks glanced at one another because they had taken vows not to touch a woman.

Then, without a word, the older monk picked up the woman, carried her across the river, placed her gently on the other side, and carried on his journey.

The younger monk couldn't believe what had just happened. After rejoining his companion, he was speechless, and an hour passed without a word between them.

Two more hours passed, then three, finally the younger monk could not contain himself any longer, and blurted out "As monks, we are not permitted a woman, how could you then carry that woman on your shoulders?"

The older monk looked at him and replied, "Brother, I set her down on the other side of the river, why are you still carrying her?"--

This simple Zen story has a beautiful message about living in the present moment. How often do we carry around past hurts, holding onto resentments when the only person we are really hurting is ourselves.

A skilled therapist will help facilitate and guide you through the emotional journey where you will discover hidden truths about your personal power. By referring to the informational categories of the Nutrient Cycle and Five Element charts, the therapist is able to trace the association of emotional traumas which register within the body causing an increase in toxic pain.

Iridology is the practice of reading the Iris to uncover weakened areas of the body which could erupt into a health crisis if not corrected. Ignatz Von Peczely 1800, originated Iridology when he discovered the correlation between a broken leg his captured Owl experienced, and the marked change in the Owl's iris relating to the broken leg. The iris can reveal energy cysts, clogged lymph and more as well.

Once these energy cysts are released they will no longer burden you and drain your energy. These sessions will help you learn to stand in your power. They will raise your level of discernment and allow you to make healthier choices going forward.

It is important to recognize the personality traits of someone with tendencies toward chronic Lyme to be those who have a penchant for rescuing others, or to be the caretaker, type A, martyr. As you release your energy cysts these self-defeating behaviors fall away and are replaced with a healthy self-respect.

You will more readily say "Yes" for *Yes* and "No" for *No*. No more people pleasing behaviors which prove to undermine all healing efforts by diverting precious energy needed for your own healing to, erroneously, be redirected to serving others who really should not be leaning on you at this time.

The full benefit of holistic therapies in the circle of life is an alchemical composite of lifestyle aspects including nutrition, work, leisure, activities, spiritual practice, associations, and stress. We have all heard stress kills. A stressful life leads to an acidic body.

The acid/alkaline balance in the blood is 7.30 - 7.45 for optimal homeostasis. We want to avoid becoming too acidic as a result of living a toxic lifestyle. Spending too much time living an acidic lifestyle full of stress, can affect our epigenetic situation and possibly eventually turn on a bad gene in our genetic code.

Instead of enabling acidic lifestyles we can turn this around by combining our understanding of the various systems of the body. Focusing on the electromagnetism of the body, along with correcting the impaired structural alignment which is creating nerve impingement, boosts our energetic stamina.

From there we can address inflammatory issues and what can be done to alleviate this damaging situation. The more we unburden our bodies from toxicity, the less pain we experience day to day.

Know your limits. Proceed with caution until you become familiar with how your body works. As you gain experience in exercising conscious manipulation over your inner-terrain, your inner-strength will grow and your pain signals will become a tool for understanding where you need to focus lifestyle clean-up efforts.

You will know you have conquered Lyme, and know you have received the benefits, when you have regained your ability to react to any given situation with measured pauses, and appropriate-sized, balanced responses based on love and gratitude. It will not be a perfect process but there is an afterthought of a job well done by defusing explosive and stressful situations which stand to confirm your healing coordinates.

SYMPATHETIC VERSUS NON-SYMPATHETIC FIGHT OR FLIGHT OR REST AND DIGEST

WELCOME TO PLANET Stress. More and more our lives seem to only get further into intensely complicated 'situations' with pressure coming at us from every angle. Watching the nightly news can devolve our spirits into the nether regions to fester. It would be prudent to consider these questions:

Why is stress such a big deal?

How does stress affect your life?

Why does perpetual stress negatively affect health and why does it need to go?

There are two systems in the body designed to help us deal with high stress and then rebalance for peaceful rest to digest aimed at rebooting our system.

The first system is the sympathetic response. Back in the day of early cave dwellers, this adrenaline rush turned on when we were in immediate danger, like running from the saber-tooth tiger. When we are faced with imminent danger our body jumps into quick action for us to either stand and fight or flee the scene. Our body, through great effort is temporarily drawing blood away from the arms and legs and pumping it directly into the heart for quick bursts of energy necessary for fighting or running. This system was only intended by Mother Nature for short energetic bursts.

Once we are out of danger the body then reverses the intense adrenaline hormonal output and returns homeostasis to a more even blood flow throughout the body. This para-sympathetic response is known as rest and digest. Now blood flows more evenly throughout the body, distributing the nutrients and oxygen for cellular nourishment and repair or sleep for restoration.

The problem with our culture today is that we are under so much stress. It seems as though we are constantly in a state of flight-or-fight/ sympathetic reaction. The high cost of this adrenaline pounding drain leads to adrenal burnout.

With kidney and adrenal burnout being the end result of chronic sympathetic stress, sadly our body has reached a state of systemic acidosis. Our preference would be to achieve a state of alkalinity as the main goal for maintaining the proper ph within the body as a result of living a balanced life.

Acid belongs in the stomach as HCL for digestion. A deficiency in certain cell salts will affect the HCL constitution resulting in digestion problems and increasing vulnerability to illness. There are significant and inexpensive tools useful for determining and adjusting an individuals cell salt imbalances which are causing these digestive systems and illness issues. Great improvements can be made by determining and correcting each individuals unique cell salt constitution.

The rest of the body needs to be alkaline which protects the organs from degeneration. When we are to acidic, the body lays down visceral fat as a protective layer to protect the organs from dissolving in these perpetual internal systemic acidic baths. This visceral fat is the toughest fat to loose when dieting because it is our inner first aid remedy. Switching to an alkaline diet will do wonders to loose weight and regain health and vitality.

We become too acidic when our lymphatic system, being the sewage system of the body which cleans out cellular debris by filtering through the kidneys and skin, gets thick with sludge and backs up toxins in the body. If our kidneys are impaired due to stress and our skin is clogged due to unhealthy lifestyle habits, the lymphatic system backs up with waste and this creates a systemic acidosis condition. Remember again, Lyme likes acidic environments. This is the main issue associated with all chronic illness.

Detoxing is the word of the day. Many concentrate on detoxing the blood through cleansing the liver and gallbladder. This is usually accomplished in 3-7 days. But when we are dealing with Lymphatic detoxing cleanses, these usually take a full 3-4 months to run a complete cycle. Parathyroid, thyroid, kidneys, and adrenals would all be working at maximum high efficiency once the lymphatic system is cleared of dehydrated mucus sludge.

Therefore, an increase in systemic acidosis along with misaligned physical body structure, leads to a complete imbalance within our body and its ability to have a strong immune system. The longer we ignore pain, override it, and press on with a "no pain, no gain" attitude, the more damage we create and the more difficult the efforts to repair and rebalance will be.

Eventually the misalignment of the bony structure, which places undue pressure on the nerves myelin sheath, will begin to shred the nerve, leading to permanent damage. One insult and injury upon another leads us down a path of aches and pains each and everyday. We become exhausted and depleted trying to override and compensate for our perpetual misalignment.

Modern life requires extra awareness of balance in life. When we trace our personal history back through our personal pain path, we begin to discover the key elements leading to our personal healing. Expanding and working our way back through the ups and downs of these issues, we stretch and grow back into our effortless state of grace.

THE GAME OF LIFE AND HOW TO PLAY IT

AS A FULL-TIME massage therapist I was wonderfully physically fit at 51. I loved my life and my work and felt fulfilled and on point. I had a bounce in my step and a sparkle in my eye. I ate right, did yoga, walked, spent time in nature, meditated but when Lyme came out of the blue and just crippled my entire life I was dumbfounded.

During the first phase I got super-skinny. Then after years in bed and unable to take care of myself and eat my healthy foods, I blew up like a tick. I gained so much weight I could only wear my sweatpants and pjs. Lyme took such a complete and devastating toll on my body and destroying my high-functioning life, that I landed in bed for nearly five years, forced to rely on family and friends just to survive.

Lyme was welcome no more. I was determined to get my health back in order. Nothing fit in my life anymore! Not my clothes, my thoughts, my friends — basically my entire life was turned inside out. I wondered to myself, *How and why did this happen?* What was the message for me behind this suffering? Always on the lookout for making sure I did not take a victim stance in my life, but rather choosing to be a Victor over all stress and strife, I knew there was a higher purpose to this sudden turn of events.

But where to start? Of course where everyone starts, with allopathic medicine. These well meaning doctors are just as frustrated as we are at the ineffective ability of the present medical care protocols for curing this devastating disease. Gratefully, due to my years of holistic healing work, I recognized there was a much more complicated healing journey ahead of me. It was going to require a complete overhaul of my entire lifestyle starting with the most basic steps such as evaluating who I was encountering in my everyday life. One of the gifts here is that you get to see who your real friends are. It is also a wonderful opportunity for people to right some wrongs in past relationships. That is some powerful healing right there.

So many of us have suffered past traumas which have resulted in an impaired ability to maintain healthy relationships. Some of us collect energy vampires around us who are people who just suck our energy for their personal gain. They talk for hours about all their problems without ever asking how you are doing. Or perhaps we were abused at some point in our past and have a self-protecting behavior of placating aggressive people in our lives, whereby, we walk on eggshells to prevent the next blowup. The reasons can be many but the results have us attracting people in our life that recreate these traumas for us on a subconscious level, over and over again, in a seemingly endless loop of draining drama.

Being that chronic Lyme suffers have personality traits of people pleasing, rescuing, caregiving, type A personalities, these relationships are a valuable source for review and change to facilitate our recovery. God, prayer, self-love and self-compassion allow us to evolve and come from a heart-centered place of awareness. Some people must go. Overtime, you will see when you ask for help who really shows up to give back and support your needs.

There are many more layers and complexities to a full recovery when dealing with these types of individuals. These are some of the essential components for laying a strong foundation on which to base recovery and a reorganized life after recovery.

Moving beyond these external sources of relationship, we travel deeper within to examine the invisible relationship we have with the invading Lyme spirochetes. As a healer I recognized the damaging affects that were resulting from this 'all out war' against Lyme disease with aggressive antibiotics.

After all, this is a God-created living being with a purpose and a will to live just as we have. The laws of karma entered the picture for me knowing I would 'get back what I put out'. If I was detonating nuclear bombs inside my gut with a constant barrage of antibiotics, I was going to pay a very high price. Mostly in the form of lost probiotic colonies, some of which would never be replaced within my gut when all was said and done.

I reasoned if the antibiotic approach was the absolute final guarantee that Lyme would be cured, then I would have to be on board. But, it became clear to me that this was not going to be the final outcome.

The antibiotics were merely a bandaid. When I was using them, I would feel somewhat better. When I was off them I was sick all over again. I needed a better way. Something that incorporated the God Force within all living things.

I decided to imagine I was playing a game of chess with Lyme as my opponent. I created a strategy whereby I would outsmart my Lyme opponent, who is really just another creature in God's kingdom. Through my focused research I found out where it lived, why it chose that location, and what damage it was doing. What were its strongholds and where were its weaknesses?

Once I had determined those statistics, I went about systematically creating an environment that would reverse the fortune Lyme spirochetes found in me as a host.

IS IT A HERXHEIMER, A HEALING CRISIS OR AM I GETTING WORSE?

AS I STARTED my research and tried different healing tools and modalities, I began to discover patterns in my healing experience. I noticed significant differences between my regular administering of healing tools like the Zapper versus prolonged periods off my program protocol which could be measured by an increase or decrease in my pain and exhaustion levels.

For example I researched what type of bed I slept in, what I brushed my teeth with, mercury fillings and dental health in general, time spent on the computer exposed to EMF's, good versus bad foods, on and on. Still today I work at discovering and refining techniques for my basic protocols to bring about a more vibrant state of health. As time goes on I feel better and better each day.

Love sustained me through this disease. It is a long, lonely journey of pain, ridicule, confusion, doubt, and fear. It is a journey that is not for the faint of heart. But if one does brave it all the way to the end, there are gifts bestowed.

There is no full recovery without these finer details of inner journeying tended to. One can choose not to address them, but I have seen the rotten fruits of denying this labor and they are quite ugly.

How long can you afford to wait to complete this healing journey? No doubt it has already come at a high cost. But view this as a gift. A chance to review and renew all that you are doing in your life. Are you truly happy? See what needs to go, what supports your health. There are deeper questions as well — what is the ultimate purpose of your life and do you feel you are on track for that goal? If not, where can you make these adjustments? There is no wiggle room at this point. Lyme forces one to review all these items and in the end, you are better for it.

In the early stages of Lyme I did not know there were to be more serious times ahead of me, including brain seizures. There was one of which sent me tumbling down the stairs resulting in contorting my foot so severely that I was not able to walk on it normally for months.

Thankfully today I have no more brain seizures, and my foot did eventually heal with lots of self-massage, energy healing and rest. Normally I would have gone right to the emergency room for such an injury. But my new fear of the medical community and their inability to cure Lyme caused me to vow never to return if possible, compound fractures aside. I cared for and nurtured my badly damaged foot with homeopathic remedies and massage, along with my holistic energetic healing skills. When my chiropractor saw the damage, he was dismayed and I think doubtful I would have a successful recovery without medical intervention. Today my foot is fine.

I will say that my best medical healing results were consistently received through chiropractic care. Not all chiropractors are alike and fortune smiled upon me with one of the best. There was yet another time of extreme body malfunction when vertigo descended upon me like a tornado out of the blue. The room spun wildly at the slightest attempt to raise my head. Even when I was lying flat the room whirled around out of control striking terror within me.

Unable to walk unassisted, I had my daughter drive me to the chiropractors office. Another grave look came upon his face as I vomited into the wastebasket in his office and apologizing, saying, "I realize this is probably outside your scope of practice ......blechhh..." But he held steady and calm as I spasmed and retched again. He checked my eyes and other evaluations to determine the root cause. I needed the lights low due to extreme sensitivity. Next he checked my walking: I was weakened but not stumbling.

Finally, after passing those tests I lay on the table and received a quick chiropractic treatment which worked to stop the vertigo. Still shaky but much relieved, I returned home to rest in bed. Each episode of extreme and explosive new symptoms opened a new chapter in determining my strategy in my game of chess with Lyme. Vertigo was to be no different.

Back in the matrix of researching healing tools to counterbalance challenging living conditions, I realized I was sleeping on a metal daybed that was acting like a virtual antenna for EMFs. This was an important revelation because EMFs make spirochetes grow. I discovered grounding habits which were to become a daily activity and yielded positive results.

Grounding while I slept and while I worked on the computer helped relieve the great muscle aches, arthritis and neuralgia which developed at the bottom of my feet years into the disease. To ground I slept on a cotton sheet with silver threads woven throughout and a cord that attached the sheet to the grounding plug in the wall socket. I learned that even if your nightstand light is turned off it is still giving off EMF frequencies.

When working on the computer I use a rubber pad which has a cord that attaches to the grounding wall socket as well. When I am outdoors I walk with bare feet on Mother Earth. The goal is to align the negative ions in the body. You know you need to get grounded when you get a shock touching a door handle and such while inside.

The biggest healing revelation came when I learned about mercury fillings and how spirochetes use heavy metals to form a protective shell called a biofilm which guards the spirochetes against medications in the blood. Dr. Landerman, DDS, has an interview entitled <u>How Lyme Hides in the Teeth</u>.

He is the original dentist to unravel the mystery of why he was not recovering from Lyme. He states that once a tooth has a filling, its integrity to self-regulate cleansing is compromised. The mouth no longer has an alkaline environment fit to tackle bacteria. Lyme spirochetes can move in and remain unchecked.

That research led me to the decision to have all amalgam fillings removed, plus a gold crown of mixed metals. This crown was over a root-canal stub and had been acting like a battery since 1972.

With the removal of all amalgam fillings and the gold mixed-metal crown, I immediately felt as if they had taken an iron mask off my head. I did experience severe herxing for one day following the procedure due to the intensity of my disability from Lyme. I did not care! I wanted to be well so much that, in the end, it was well worth the effort. I followed this dental work with several sessions of acupuncture to balance my meridians.

Please note that choosing the right dentist is essential. Not all dentists who claim they are biological dentists are specialists in removing mercury fillings. Call and inquire to be sure they are using protective dams, masks, provide extra oxygen and have a special air vacuum to remove the mercury particles released into the air during this procedure. When these alma gam fillings are removed, they are considered Hazardous Waste and must be disposed of according to environmental laws.

On and on went my recovery. I would have one step forward, then two, and then a setback would emerge. Through it all I just kept taking baby steps, doing the next thing in front of me.

Eventually the time began to add up and compound. There was no standalone tool, no "one size fits all" solution. Instead, there was an emphasis on a certain order of tools and changes to my lifestyle habits.

Some tools would advance my healing quickly. Other treatments did nothing. I did not judge tools or treatments. I just tried them and at the appropriate times moved on.

It is a multi-faceted journey that can take years depending on how disciplined one is with following healing protocols. No, it was not easy. Praying everyday and keeping faith in God as the universal source is crucial.

> "It is not the food in your life that counts,
> but the life in your food that nourishes."
>
> —Dr. Aris Latham

Nutrition is of the utmost importance. It is vital to incorporate non-inflammatory foods along with energetically harmonious foods to guide us to supreme health.

We are what we eat. If the animal we are consuming has had a wonderful life, was grass-fed and free-roaming, then that being will have good hormonal resonance.

If it has had a life of imprisonment, violence, and GMO grains instead of its natural diet, then this animal will have hateful, violent, fear-based hormonal baths flooding their tissue. When we consume this negative energy, it becomes part of our cellular structure. Perhaps this is part of the reason society seems to be so far off track now. It is something to consider.

Following the health and nutrition laws in the Bible can be very much a part of this journey as well. Laws such as not eating shrimp, lobster, and shellfish—all crustaceans—because they are scavengers provide powerful awareness. Pork is also a no-no. Pigs do not have sweat glands; therefore, they do not eliminate toxins. When we eat the flesh of these creatures, we are filled with this garbage and toxic sludge. God has provided all the guidance we need with food sources, healing oils, prayer life, moral construct. I find so many are so quick to jump all over Scripture without ever having researched and applied it to their own life with an open heart. You are what you eat, think, feel and breathe.

Parasites are thought to play a role in Lyme. Pork, for example, can harbor some of the most deadly parasites that will not be destroyed, even at the highest temperatures of 400 degrees and more. It has been found that parasites can lead to disease, mood rages, and general health. Removal of parasites must be done slowly and with great care.

As I stated before, there are many caring doctors attempting to treat Lyme who are just as frustrated as we are at the ineffective treatments and funding for further research. I was disappointed with the endless doctor visits, having had more than a few negative standout experiences. I feel it is important to state here that I had always, up until then, had a very positive experience with doctors. All my past medical needs had been met with compassion and skilled caring. I just assumed it would be the same for Lyme disease, but that was not the case. This disease is a true mystery that takes time to unravel.

I was introduced to herbal tinctures on various occasions and found them to be a powerful substitute for antibiotic treatment. I did not combine herbal tinctures with antibiotic use because the frequencies of herbal tinctures are much more refined and delicate compared to the heavy handed antibiotic medications.

I used Teasel root to control the behavior of the spirochetes. Teasel root is an invasive weed brought in by Mother Nature for this burgeoning epidemic which I found to be the perfect remedy to coax the stubborn spirochete out of their hiding places they had burrowed into. I followed that revelation with another powerful invasive weed made into a tincture called Japanese Knotweed which is a natural antibiotic loaded with Resveratrol.

The key to optimizing effective use of these tinctures was to be consistent with administration, yet varying the timing by five or ten minutes to keep the spirochetes guessing. I did not ingest disharmonious pharmaceuticals and removed all fluoride from my water, including bath and shower water.

I committed to using the tinctures daily for 3-4 months without judging my recovery. I just prayed over the bottles and kept the faith they would work. And yes they did! Once I felt the healing relief start to emerge from these tinctures I then added herbal teas such as Cats Claw, Pau d'Arco, Blessed Thistle, Wormwood. I also added adaptive medicinal mushrooms and then superfoods to my treatment plan. Experiencing these promising results I decided to continue on with their usage until I was sure Lyme was conquered.

I still use these products today in a more relaxed and enjoyable manner. I will make sun teas with the herbs and adaptive mushrooms. I make elixirs with the superfoods and use the teas as a base. Their nutritional benefit extends well beyond just the properties of healing Lyme and co-infections.

As I work in the garden these days I take great precaution not to get re-bitten but there is the occasional event where I find a tick attached. I remove the tick properly first by placing a tick key at the mouth of the tick and twirl the tick key and lift the tick off. I swab the area with hydrogen peroxide or turpentine. Then I immediately head for the kitchen cabinet and take doses of Andrographis, Teasel root and Japanese Knotweed for several days until I am sure I am out of danger. I also run extra session with my far infra red sauna and enemas.

One bite last year gave me an exposure to bartonella even with all the added remedies. I will say that infection could have raged on for a year or more but with diligence, I was able to overcome the painful experience within four months. Prevention is still the best cure!

Recovery will take time, but there will be the day when you draw back to observe the situation and recognize that you *are* making progress. Things are starting to shift in a good direction. There will be setbacks of various kinds of course as you move along, but they will be fewer and fewer as you become stronger and stronger.

During the disease you will experience the Herxheimer reactions which may include: runny nose, hiccups, loose stools, gas, bloating, vomiting, heartburn, fatigue, flushing, sleep disturbance, burping, blisters, chills, nausea, flatulence, and cold sores. These will all go away slowly as you keep working at eliminating lifestyle behaviors which empower the spirochete.

These have been some of my Lyme healing highlights. There were many more times of crying for days on end, vomiting wildly for days on end and excruciating headaches. I couldn't imagine how I could endure any more pain beyond what was delivered.

There were mysterious rashes and deep chronic fatigue so bad I felt that sleeping for one hundred years would not be enough. All this was accompanied by fibromyalgia pain inflaming and encompassing soft tissue throughout my body.

Other times I endured bone-gnawing pain that twisted so deeply it would steal my breath away. I felt like the disease was literally eating the flesh off my bones. For years on end this was my everyday experience, shut up in a bed, writhing in pain and agony, screaming, crying, and dying in pain. No one had answers, only roadblocks, sarcasm, denials, and arrogance. My heart was broken.

How do I tell you that there were experiences so cruel on the part of the insurance company that you have to wonder if they were, in fact, at all human? I cannot even bring myself to put into print what I endured at their lack of mercy.

Eventually the doctors reports said I would never work again. If I stayed on that same trajectory, they were right. I decided to take matters into my own hands and see what I could do to recover according to the laws of Mother Nature and common sense.

I prayed and God answered. I had to learn to quiet my mind and my life enough to hear the guidance laid out for you here in these pages.

Today I live a wonderful life full of health and vitality. The changes made in my life accommodating my full recovery are now my everyday habits and holistic self-care routines. When my mindfulness and adherence to these healthful strategies stray too far from my core protocol, as happens occasionally, I feel the effects of toxicity creeping back in. It is important to note there that these feelings of relapse are not active Lyme but rather the symptoms of toxic lifestyle building up within my system. You will learn the difference as you heal.

Lyme damaged my body and I am very sensitive to environmental stimulants. But since my recovery I will say nothing resembles the level of pain and illness of active Lyme disease. When I start to feel the effects of toxic lifestyle and nutrition, I simply apply the protocol more diligently and it all disappears within a very short period of time. Lyme disease left damage in its wake, but thankfully I am now returning to a outstanding healthy status. Better than ever.

I work everyday to do at least one therapeutic modality so I will continue to improve. Today I shine! I still study to learn some new wonder about the human body and its capability to self-heal. Now it is for my personal enjoyment rather then in desperation to heal. I have discovered it seems we would do well to get out of our own way and let the body's self-healing capability emerge on its own.

> "Populations problems have a horrible
> way of solving themselves."
>
> —Robert Hienman

10 STEP PROTOCOL FOR LYME DISEASE AND CO-INFECTIONS

TO UNDERSTAND SOMETHING is to be liberated from it. The biggest question I am asked is based on the fact that you can know all the right things to do but if you do not do them in the right order, they will not work. Everyone wants to know "What is the right order?". This order is based on your personal history relating to your present state of health, lifestyle and nutritional habits, emotional balance and spiritual foundation. Each segment will have its own set of ordered criteria.

As we inventory and examine what you are presently doing which will lead to your recovery from chronic Lyme disease and co-infections, our goal is to develop an alternative plan beyond struggling with antibiotics.

Remembering this is not a war against Lyme and co-infections but rather a strategic play in this game of life hologram, we acquire a desire to develop strategies used in the game of chess. We imagine two opponents concentrating and planning moves designed to knock the other out of power.

At first it can look like one side is winning, only to then have that side become submerged due to underestimating their opponents skill and strategy. Other times there is a take back of ground whereby a sudden and unexpected surge promotes the other, toward getting the upper hand, with a sweeping victory.

This winning strategic competition will necessitate thoughtful and cautious thinking ahead by several moves, while assessing the risks for each move taken. This involves a wider view to include, as much as is possible, all possible outcomes involved.

Impulsive actions with no future planning could be very risky, therefore, allowing the opponent to take advantage of the situation. It can be difficult to relax into this give-and-take process in the beginning. At times we will feel defeated and frustrated as the struggle seems to go on and on.

The goal is to remain focused and concentrate on the main outcome. Methodical, step-by-step moves with wisdom, purpose and forward thinking will save the day and, ultimately, win your vitality and joy back.

Our choices should be guided by what makes our life sweeter, easier, more joyful, productive and healthy. We want a purpose driven life, to be a team player, with clean and lively energy.

1) Mindset: Lyme and co-infections are very tricky little beings who have a will to survive all their own. We become the host. *In this impersonal internal game of strategy and intrigue, we start with the mindset that all of life is vibration.* This vibration is created by thought and light which eventually manifests into the physical when held in focus long enough through the Chakra system. We begin with the smallest point of clarity: the name of the disease. It is officially 'Lyme,' not 'Lymes'. Focusing on such a point might not impress most people but each should reconsider that such details are an important concept carried throughout all healing journeys in general. In the end Lyme is an energetic vibrational recalibration of the hosts nervous system, physical and mental structure, and spiritual vibration. This challenging and painful journey results in an elevation of the hosts overall energetic wellbeing when addressed at these levels. Even the spasmodic restless muscle twitches in legs and body, similar to shaking a rag doll, these parts can be calmed, mastered and used to our benefit through aligned meditational insight. Nestling into weakened and injured areas within our body, Lyme reveals the keys to unlocking our personal history mystery. Ultimately Lyme and company may put a calling on our life requiring us

to play a bigger game. Start to incorporate the tools and steps that speak to you as you become more attuned to your own living vibration through focused mindset. Once familiar with your own pure personal vibration, move forward by comparing your vibration to that of the spirochetes during their invading cycled expansion. Sensitivity to these subtle energies will take time to develop. Everyone has this gift.

2) Have a Heart Safe Harbor of strong network support with the most uplifting and positive people you can call on during the days and nights when this disease kicks you down and tears you up. Please remember to reach out for help. Select carefully those of your inner circle. This is a time when you will find out who your real friends are. Use discernment in choosing between the two types of people in the world. Those known as energy vampires who selfishly syphon off our goodness, versus those who give us heart-centered healing energy from their own open hearts. Pray for guidance and for help from spirit in all these matters. This is your time to change any self-sabotaging people-pleasing behaviors and habits which may have a role in chronic illness and disease playing out in your life today.

3) Clean pure living vibrational water is essential to healing. Working with the brilliant genius of Viktor Schauberger (1885-1958), who possessed a deep understanding of the role of the Divine in Natures evolutionary process, we regard water as a sacred organism. It becomes clear that spring water, with low TDS, is the most vibrant solution. Divine water empowers our living body through maturation of water molecules which then levitate up to the surface. That is how a tree is watered in nature, not by sucking water up from the ground up but, rather, through levitation. Vibrant water is also ideal for dissolving the pollution and stagnation within our blood, lymph and interstitial fluid systems. This congestion concentrates toxicities and suppresses our immune system, keeping it from optimal function. Spring water is water that has been allowed to ripen, versus, well water being prematurely drawn up or municipal water laden with many contaminants, which cannot be processed out. Ripe

spring water has sweetness from carbohydrates which well water and tap water do not contain.

4) Clean air and deep abdominal breathing seem simple enough when you live in the country, but if you live near a city or commute in heavy traffic, you are more likely going to be exposed to mold and toxins on a consistent basis. If you suspect mold get tests to confirm what you are up against. When you see spraying of chemicals in the air, go inside and close all windows and doors until the spraying has stopped. For the breathing exercises, set aside some quiet time, even if it is just for a few moments. You may lay down with as little pillow as possible, shoes off and belts loosened; or, you may sit in a chair with your back straight and away from the wall or back of chair, hips rolled forward. As you begin breathing allow your belly to soften and expand,; allow the diaphragm to distend into the abdominal region. Expand up into the chest cavity by building gently upon the abdominal breath. Focus on bringing the energy up into the lungs; expand through the shoulders and sternum with a gentle flexing arch extension of the thoracic and cervical spine. Next, expand this in breath to the top of the head. HOLD at the top of the breath for a count of four. Then gently begin to EXHALE, as if blowing out a candle, all the way to empty lungs. At this point there are two different methods of breathing. *One will invite sympathetic, fight or flight response and the other will induce a para-sympathetic, rest and digest response.* The sympathetic breathing response will be charged up when we EXHALE for a count of four, then HOLD at the bottom of this EXHALE for a count of four. This *stop-and-hold action* of the EXHALE actually stresses the body and provokes a high-alert status. Whereas, if one wants to induce rest and digest para-sympathetic response, the key is to allow and follow each EXHALE to continue all the way to the very end of each EXHALE. You just keep blowing out and blowing out, and blowing out, even into sputtering. When all the air is out, gently REVERSE the air flow by releasing the EXHALE and gently begin to INHALE. The continual flow

of one stream of one into another, then gently back into itself, will allow you to relax deeper and deeper into quiet meditation.

5) Sunshine and sun soaks are another hot topic. Sunshine directly onto our skin facilitates the production of Vitamin D whose main function is to promote calcium absorption in the body. Through the eyes sun shine stimulates the pituitary gland in the brain along with the hypothalamus gland which affects our circadian rhythm. Limited exposure is the key to health and vitality sun soaking. During the late 19th and early 20th centuries, tuberculosis was the leading cause of death in the United States. Consequently, the most popular and widely accepted treatments involved clean air, low humidity, cool nights, and abundant sunshine. By the late 1800s, "Sanitariums," designated and built in various temperate locations throughout the country, would roll the patients in their beds out onto the veranda for therapeutic sun soaks. Remember to employ commonsense and respect for the power of the sun which is strongest and hottest between 10 am and 2 pm. The fairer you are the more cautious you want to be as you monitor your sun exposure. Avoid chemical sunscreens. The beneficial sun is blocked when we wear sunglasses, contact lenses, glasses and are behind windows. Healthy skin will not burn if it is full of collagen, elastic and properly maintained with dry skin brushing, deep cleansing, saunas and by consuming certain sun protective foods.

6) Detox and Rejuvenation keep our body exits clear for bringing out the trash post-cellular metabolism. Blood is the kitchen delivering nutrients and oxygen; Lymph is the sewage system carrying the garbage to the exit zones of the kidneys, bladder, lungs and skin. If our liver and gallbladder are full of toxins they cannot properly aid in maintaining the blood; if the kidneys, lungs and skin are clogged they cannot aid in properly maintaining the lymph. Blood is 1/3 of the body fluid and lymph is 2/3 of the total body fluid content. Imagine if your sink and toilet were clogged with bacon fat and grease and yet, you kept putting waste into them, flushing and waiting for the vessel to empty. It is just not going to happen. Eventually everything

backs up and overflows. This is how hardened lymphatic vessels develop. To reverse this issue, detox all the eliminative organs through supervised nutritional juicing, herbs or fasting. Consult your LD primary care practitioner before undertaking any new cleansing diets.

7) Nutrition and lifestyle are key components. This is not a quick fix system. It is rather an all encompassing lifestyle protocol realignment. Subjecting oneself to self-imposed discipline is the surest way to increase the quality of ones existence. If you are going to live longer you want the highest healthiest quality of life. Being that our world is so toxic these days from our water to our air to our food, it is evermore important to choose organic foods, clean high-vibration water, low EMF's, strong boundaries. It is a daily awareness and best achieved slowly with particular attention to proper nutrients, eating times, exercise styles, detoxing, energetics of people you are involved with, work environment and so on. Many people demand from me a list, in correct order, which they can follow all up front. This is not entirely useful. Some do not want to hear that everyone is different and that each item must be examined, weighed and measured to determine if it is having a positive or negative affect. As one becomes more closely aligned with this process it will happen faster and easier each time. One phase of alignment builds upon the next and compounds in more positive affects as we move along.

8) Restorative grounding rest is essential for prime healing. Lyme disturbs our healing sleep, awakening us at all hours, as the spirochetes grow. Symptoms of painful restlessness, particularly involving the legs, is often referred to as Restless Leg Syndrome. There could be sensations of bugs crawling all over our skin such as an invisible enemy. Terror and pain wrack the body over and over, relentless writhing flesh. Hormones are out of whack. To align with better sleep habits and get out of this sleep deprivation nightmare, create a bedtime routine to shift and unplug from this surrounding noisy world. Align with a gentle sleep preparation routine by being unplugged from all

EMF exposure prior to being ready for deep and restorative bedrest. Our immune system reboots itself during 10:00 p.m. to 2:00 a.m. in the 24 hour sleep cycle. If you miss that time slot in the evening, the time slot of 10:00 a.m. to 2:00 p.m. will also work. Anchor yourself quietly. Let your wisdom flow. Let stress melt away. Our culture is chronically out in the world banging on delicate adrenals with stimulants such as coffee, cigarettes, stress. We can use our intentional resting time to receive relaxing hormone body soaks, which provide our whole physiology with quiet and peaceful vibrations. Engaging in divine joyful movement each day, even if it is just a small walk to the end of the path and back, is necessary. Do not choose aerobic, but rather, choose anaerobic exercise. Pilates, yoga, weight training, walking at your comfort level of fitness.

9) A healthy gut bio-dynamic flora energetically mimics the Tree of Life spiraling upward, expanding from the gut to the brain, one strength builds upon another. Serotonin for the brain is produced in the gut. If there are any issues involving the foundation of our existence disturbing root chakra flora, addressing these imbalances is crucial. If we are low in B vitamins or do not methylate Bs well, our nervous system is in jeopardy. Certain gut flora produce our B vitamins, B12 excluded. Consuming a methylated B12 is recommended. Eating live fermented foods is one way to increase probiotic colonies, some of which produce our B vitamins. We must address any Irritable Bowel Syndrome, mold, parasites, leaky gut, allergens, inflammation, which provoke and promote yeast overgrowth. When climbing the ladder of health success, make sure it is up against the right wall which has a strong foundation.

10) A healthy mouth equals a healthy body, hand-n-hand, mouthful-by-mouthful, check-up by check-up. Does your tongue sparkle or is it mucus coated or deeply crevassed? Alma gams, root canals, gold crowns are all contributing factors connected to longterm health status. By combining wellness know-how and self-care techniques, we enhance our immune system strength, thereby, throughly eliminating the comfy-cozy spirochete

nestling incubator coves. Mercury dental alma gams are slated to be phased out by 2020 and all mercury mining is stopping altogether. After removing alma gams and root canals when stuck in this chronic debilitating disease, my healing journey turned around. Do your research and choose a biological dentist who specializes in removing mercury. There are special procedures and equipment that go along with this procedure.

At the end of the day you have to believe in "self-response-ability" by taking control of your life and health. Balkers claim "but I *have* tried everything!". To which I say "EVERYTHING? You say you have tried EVERYTHING?"; I say "No, you have not tried *Everything!*"

Success is living joy with love through congruent integrity.

What is working for you?

What does a successful recovery look like for you?

THE GIFT OF LYME

PERHAPS YOUR WORLD spun quickly out of control once you were hit with Lyme, or you could have it stealthily lurking about with painful, surprising, frequent attacks spanning decades of your life. Life with Lyme is chaos or frequently devolves into chaos more often than not.

The goal is to quiet the internal playing field by leveling off and stopping exposure to toxicities on all fronts. Turning down the internal heat relieves inflammation and the resulting inner-terrain is clearer. When we begin to dismantle bad habits from their root causes, we have more control.

Eliminate one bad habit and then introduce a healthy recovery step to fill the void which was created from the withdrawal of said habit. For example, by reducing total coffee intake to just a.m., wean off by following up with super juice of beets, lemons, limes, greens, celery, cucumber, ginger for the rest of the day!

Support is an essential element through the roller coaster ride of recovery. Design a written, step-by-step plan for each individual situation. Guidance for refining and incorporating recovery tools is most beneficial from someone who has already walked this path you are now on and returned safely. Keep the faith that Spirit is guiding you to the next right thing.

Go deeper into reading body language to determine energy cysts embedded within the tissue that are creating blockages in the flow of chi's vital life force. With our health back on track commit to incorporate a healthier lifestyle to carry through the following decades. Reinforce new and healthy lifestyle habits daily.

Your reward is an upgraded life force energy with which to carry one forward into their destiny and life purpose. Dreams fulfilled with an appreciation far beyond what was once thought possible. The key is to never give up. Remember it is darkest right before the dawn.

PHYSICAL DETOX

HAVING DETERMINED THE need to bear down on this disease how do we begin to fight the good fight? Self-Empowerment is developed through mindfulness as the first step. We must have a can-do, failure-is-not-an-option attitude. For example, years into my research I discovered spirochetes grow at night. From there on I developed a specific strategy to not provide nourishment or energy for these colony growth spurt periods.

Everyday I learned something new to apply to my healing. Never give up. Even if you think you have tried everything, I am here to tell you that you have not tried everything. Dig deeper, again.

A healing journey incorporates the gifts and lessons accrued along the path. We will do well to follow the path of least resistance. Alignment to this path of least resistance is known by joy, ease, and happiness. Anything negative is out of alignment. There is a great back-and-forth movement along this path. When we do not follow the path of least resistance, we encounter roadblocks which serve to correct the course along this path.

We each have a unique resonance within us which we may choose to utilize as a guiding force. It is called our intuition or innate knowing. It is our third brain, our gut, which tells us 'you've got guidance'. Polish the looking glass, clear the fog from the mirror and adjust the dial.

Lyme has a longterm impact on the energetic nervous system by this constant increase of vibration. Ultimately, this exchange provides an awakened lightness of being which resonates with the rainbow bridge, thereby, allowing fuller access to the new earth 5th dimensional reality. Here we are blessed with a renewed and forgiving nature based on compassion and heart-centered love. We concentrate exclusively on our everyday choices which lead either 'toward' or 'away from' our desired state of health and vitality.

Lyme is indiscriminate in its destruction. Just because one practices a healing profession, does not grant nor guarantee asylum from life's painful lessons. We do not get extra credit by practicing spiritually, eating right, visiting spiritual places, practicing spiritual materiality or because we learn from spiritual teachers. For Lyme, everyone is fair game.

True healing is a journey into the dark night of the soul and back. It is a journey that shakes one to the core, cracking one open, ripping apart ego-based delusions, and dissolving any resistance to self-responsibility and ownership of only playing half-in the game.

Be careful what you ask for. The universe is always listening. It will grant your wishes. Your dreams will manifest. Embrace your souls divine path if you are a seeker. Call forth lessons which spark congruent integrity and endurance. True mastery cannot be discovered in a book or taught in a class. These lessons are whispering moments of alignment. Once we set our foot on the path, there is no turning back. As Betty Davis said, "Fasten your seat belt. It's going to be a bumpy ride." All is one.

Optimal healing requires the deconstruction of outmoded subconscious rigid issues from past matters, unknowingly influencing our lives, the world around us, and our place in it. We cannot divorce ourselves from the truth that we live in a world of toxic pollution, greed, plunder, betrayal and deceit. Harsh, but true.

Life is a struggle for territory, either advancing or retreating, through a series of checks and balances. We must learn discernment and trust our gut, which when balanced, taps into our inner truth.

We begin the journey of physical healing in the gut. We address the blood to enhance the distribution of nutrients and oxygen. We address the lymphatic sewage system to rid the body of toxic waste. Onward and upward we focus on maintaining a balance between our acid vs alkaline internal pH environment. We walk away from systemic acidosis.

For humans, the alimentary canal is our first line of defense against invading microbes. The intestines benefit from fiber which serves to escort harmful organisms out of the body through the colon. The small and large intestine meanwhile are filtering what we eat and drink to assimilate nutrients, minerals, vitamins, and enzymes for future cellular metabolism.

We are bombarded daily by environmental toxins beyond our control. The Chernobyl and Fukushima catastrophes together have forever elevated our exposure to radioactive nuclear contamination. Elsewhere we are bombarded with x-rays, EMF exposure through treatments, airports, wireless modems, cell phones, iPads and more.

Compound these issues with fluoride, heavy-metal poisoning from alma gam fillings, vaccines, and fish for a toxic soup. Sadly, our soil is in a state of severe mineral depletion too yielding nutritionally inferior foods. You would need to eat five apples today to match the nutritional equivalent of one of the apples our grandparents ate. Health is an everyday concern.

Today we can no longer blindly trust our food sources. We can ill afford to blindly turnover our health to medical practices without doing our own homework. We must take our power back by accepting full responsibility for our own role in our personal health and wellness.

Our health is our new Wealth. When that precious gift is gone the road back to vitality and everyday normal living is no longer guaranteed. In other words, it is easier to stay healthy than to try to recover health.

Time to step up!

EMOTIONAL DETOX

THERE IS A wonderful tool called the Ho'oponopono Prayer from Hawaii. It was used by a psychiatrist who treated prisoners in one of the states worst prison. He would take the prisoner files one at time and repeat this prayer over the files. Over time, these prisoners began turning their lives around.

Ho'oponopono Prayer

> I'm sorry
>
> Please forgive me
>
> Thank you
>
> I love you

In the beginning when doing this prayer I was shocked to find that although I thought I was forgiving people from perceived past hurts, I still had a way to go. My heart was not as light and easy as I had expected. It was instead locked up in bitterness and anger around certain circumstances. As I sat with these feelings and melted through them one at a time, I began to experience a truer healing of love, forgiveness and compassion. It was within these surrendering moments that my deeper healing from Lyme disease began to take hold.

I still use these skills today. Life is a constant roller-coaster ride of challenges and issues. If we truly embrace being here to learn life lessons for our spiritual development, just like peeling an onion, we know there is always more onion!

Meditate upon the beauty and wonder of life. Make a gratitude list each night before you go to bed. Live the way you expect wellness would feel. No second guessing, no thinking you are not worthy. Be sure to take time for your emotional examination and shift in perspectives where necessary.

SPIRITUAL DETOX

MEDITATION AND VISUALIZATION of a healing energetic imprint will direct your focus to the higher enjoyment of life without struggle. Relax and completely let the mind chatter go. Allow complete mind meditation to ripple down the spine. Allow your extremities to relax. Allow slower, deeper more purposeful breathing. Allow inspiration to arise from the darkness.

Like a phoenix rising from the ashes rest long enough to revitalize. Tap off any energy leaks you have found during your quiet rest. Allow forgiveness to manifest instantly. This complex game of healing has something to teach. It is through our choices, especially during moments we think no one is looking and really everyone is looking, that our destiny is shaped. Spirit watches all the time.

Try this experiment: Sit quietly for a moment and center yourself. Breathe in through your nose. See the air swirl through the bone at the top of your nose which creates a vortex driving air into the deepest regions of your lungs. Hold for a count of four. Then exhale through your mouth as if you are blowing out a candle. Repeat gently and rhythmically.

Now think of an issue, a person, or situation which causes you anxiety. Feel where that goes in your body.

How does that affect your breath, your heart, and your muscles?

Is your jaw clenched?

Does your breathing rate increase?

Do you feel anger and want to get back into the offending situation or do you want revenge?

Feel these issues as you sit deeper and deeper into your helplessness, your tears, and your vulnerability.

Now center into your heart and feel the tension build. Then repeat to yourself, "I am letting this go and letting this go, and I am letting this go." As each thought rises up repeat the phrase "I am letting this go....".

Each time you repeat the phrase to yourself, feel your heart lighten, expand, and open. As you turn your anger over to the Divine, your heart space will open and expand freely in all directions.

The tension will melt away more and more each time you repeat the "letting go" phrase. Perhaps you can do this ten times or fifteen times. Then rest quietly and feel the lightness of your heart.

As you discover deeper layers of resistance ask yourself quietly what could the matter be? It is hard not to blame others for something you know they should have done to help you but did not. No excuses, right? But we are all human. Who of us has done something we know we could have done better? We all have.

People are merely a mirror of what we like or dislike about ourselves that we see in them reflecting back to us. Remember we get back what we put out. To stay angry at someone is self destructive. Meanwhile, they have gone on to live a happy life totally unaware of our angst, suffering, and wasteful lust for revenge.

What about when there is the matter of congruent integrity? The other person should have not lied and betrayed you. They should own up to their mistake or said they were sorry. Here we must be the change we want to see in the world. We must make a conscious decision and choose our measured and balanced reaction based on compassion, forgiveness and love.

We must not let our E. G. O. (Edge God Out) rule the day. It is okay to step up, swallow our pride, and be the first to forgive. Miracles happen.

WALK INTO GRACE

THE GLOVES ARE off and the game is on! Are you willing to do whatever it takes to overcome this illness? There is a gift at the end of the journey bestowed upon those who apply themselves through acceptance, surrender and never quit.

To be engulfed with a full-time disability is an enormous education. To be divided from one's health for years upon years is truly a rugged experience for the soul. What is the goal? Why are we here, and how do we get back to joy and health?

Do not argue with life. See it for what it is. You will know you are on the right path to wellness when you will feel it begin to emerge in your body. You will feel ripples at first of peace, calm, relaxation, openness, easy breathing, energy, and core strength and finally gratitude.

The healing work is incremental, each day adding a touch more support in green foods, medicinal mushrooms, cleansing fruits, healing tonics, elixirs, lifestyle, and habit overhaul. Start with clean water. To build a house you must have a strong foundation. To heal it is the same; the foundation is where we start. Please take this into your heart. You will gain the upper-hand, and your recovery will accelerate greatly. Lose the resistance. Nurture and protect your inner sanctum with strategy rather than creating a battlefield filled with harsh anti-biotic anxiety.

These letting-go episodes will be experienced at different paces and to different degrees. Sometimes one release is all we will have. Other times, it is like a kaleidoscope of Technicolor flashback memories spewing for hours on end while the liver painfully cramps and convulsively repeatedly expels bile. Liver is where we store anger. Hold that space of Love and Forgiveness until the pain subsides.

Trust that your body knows this process of letting go. There is no need to keep score; just observe as tension melts away. With active Lyme there is no strength for fighting back. Let the anxiety wash over you and drain away the pain bit by bit until your body falls limp again and again.

It is all part of our unfolding and stepping into the light.

> *Our struggles with life and anxiety blockages aids us in the process by building up agitated tension, which is then the catalyst that facilitates this letting-go process.*

Like a balloon full of air, each time we process letting go evenly and with control, the less inner tension we have to endure and the more peaceful our walk.

Ancient healing traditions of Upanishads see Stars inside our hearts, which help us to see with our hearts, and to heal with our hearts radiant light.

OPENING TO YOUR OWN HEALING POTENTIAL

UPSTATE NEW YORK is tick territory! When I attend the local Lyme support meetings it is heartbreaking to hear the stories of suffering. I offer all the remedies and tools designed by Mother Nature that I used for curing myself from Lyme but surprisingly many people resist incorporating even the simplest of these remedies.

They search for answers. They pound on doctors desks demanding a cure, all the while missing the elements we are discussing here. Give yourselves a big hug and recognize you are the ones doing the real work!

Action is what counts. Taking action and never giving up! I respect you all very much for taking this journey.

So frustrating! Really! It is beginning to seem like we can look forward to Lyme, now a Green Ribbon event, being a long-time mystery disease to be unraveled. When I finally accepted that the doctors did not have the answer for my cure, I realized I needed to step up and take matters into my own hands.

I finally did win the battle. It was a lifestyle makeover including a new level of awareness around nutrition, relationships, lymph and blood detoxing, sunshine, water, tinctures, saunas, enemas, and dental work. One thing after another helped me move closer to the sparkling wellness I enjoy today.

Research is always essential for selecting the best tools to meet individual goals and needs. Being nearly homeless and unable to work due to full Lyme disability, I was highly motivated to design a most cost-efficient program. Body-map reading reveals keys to unlocking the mystery.

Lyme puts a calling on our life requiring we play a bigger game. I encourage you to incorporate those tools which speak to you.

We are here to transmute these difficulties into the highest and best good using uplifting, positive energy. On days when this disease kicks us down, please reach out for help. Everyone has a gift of perspective. The only people who were truly able to help me were the people who had experienced Lyme personally.

There are some who use bee-sting therapy to heal. Back then I only had enough energy to do what was exactly in front of me and which came together easily. I constantly modified my lifestyle, nutrition, and inner terrain and incorporated herbs.

Recently, as I have been working in the yard I actually have received a bunch of bee stings! Whaaa! I run in and grab the baking soda, mix it with water to make a paste and slap it on the sting. It immediately calms the situation and I like to think I get the benefit of the sting too based on Mother Nature's timing wisdom. I bless the bee who gave its life for my wellness. Everything always comes back around to a blessing. It works!

At one point during my inability to overcome Lyme, I realized that this situation was bigger than myself. I accepted it finally as an assignment from God the Universal Source.

These were the actual steps I used to turn my situation around. I hit the reset button and untangled this mystery like a cat after a ball of yarn.

After I was blessed with the grace of healing, I felt the need to assist others in my own humble way. I hold the vision that all will be well. Lives will return to a healthy, vibrant flow. I pray the gift of this disease be revealed to each in Divine timing as it is in alignment with each energetic vibration for the Highest and Best Good.

FREQUENTLY ASKED QUESTIONS

Q. What should I do to protect against being reinfected?

A. Time is of the essence when dealing with Lyme disease. Prevention is the best cure. I always keep bottles of Andrographis, Teasel root, and Japanese knotweed tinctures in the cabinet.

WHENEVER I HAVE been gardening or if I find a tick on me, I immediately remove the tick properly by holding the tick mouth. Be careful not to squeeze contents of the ticks stomach into host when removing it. If the tick is already embedded, I swab it with turpentine on a Q-tip. You can actually feel the tick die following this application.

Then I place a dropper of Andrographis under my tongue three times a day for three days. We have the best chance of warding off the disease with immediate action. Spirochetes live for approximately eight to eleven days in the bloodstream before they spiral their way into areas like bone, organs and the like to hide where medication cannot go.

A warning note about Andrographis.

Some people have experienced a severe rash from the use of Andrographis. Approximately one percent of people experience a rash, most often like hives, which can cover much of the body. It will clear by discontinuing Andrographis. It can take up to a month for this to clear. The scientific literature on Andrographis notes potential allergic reaction. Caution should be exercised. If you do experience an allergic reaction, discontinue use of this herb. After the rash has cleared, you may reintroduce the herb carefully at low doses.

Q. What is the best way to get vitamin D?

A. With limited skin-to-sunshine exposure. I personally do not use creams or sunscreen lotions. I rather choose to sit in the sun and have my skin soak up direct rays from the sun. These rays on our skin interact with cholesterol to make hormones. Some sunscreens contain chemicals that are harmful. Common sense should prevail for exposure times. I usually sit for twenty minutes each day.

Sunglasses are also a hindrance to receiving the benefits from the sun rays. This is a tough one, because Lyme makes our eyes so sensitive to light. Each sunny day I sit facing the sun, eyes closed, with no sunglasses, for a beautiful sun-soak healing.

Q. How can I address the pins-and-needles feeling and pain on the bottom of my feet?

A. Grounding is fun and easy. Some feel this disconnection from nature's rhythm is due to EMFs disrupting our entire energy field. Rubber soles on our shoes and sneakers cut us off from the earth's ionic alignment.

The solution: take your shoes off and stand on the earth to ground your energy by realigning your negative ions. This is also known to ease jet lag when you stand on the new time zone land with bare feet.

Another source of neuropathy is lack of B vitamins. Check to see if you are methylating B vitamins and consider methylated B-12. Also consider consuming live fermented foods or probiotics to enhance gut flora.

Q. What is one main concept for healing from Lyme?

A. It's amazing how much pain and destruction accompanies these nasty diseases. The state of the body should be one of pain-free health and vitality. We need to look within and modify our inner-terrain, going from a state of systemic acidosis to a state of alkalinity.

Q. How long will it take to heal from Lyme?

A. The answer is different for everyone. Healing is now your full-time job. Put the oxygen mask on yourself first. You can know all the right things to do, but if you do not do them in the right order, they will not work. Mindset is first on the list.

Q. What is the role of the Lyme corkscrew spirochete in nature?

A. Mother Nature employs the corkscrew spirochetes design to make deer antlers grow. We are one part of a complete world with mysteries we may never solve.

Q. What role does mercury alma gam fillings play in disease and recovery?

A. Cleaning up the mercury is one of the best strategic tools. Regarding composites, Dr. Landerman, DDS, of Sebastol, California, recommends body-testing each individual by a qualified biological dentist to see which replacement composite is preferable for his or her body type. My gold tooth crown over a root canal was discovered to have "gold" mixed metals and was acting like a battery. It was a case of double trouble, as the root-canal stub was a breeding ground for bacteria since only the main root nerve can be extracted, beyond that there are thousands of tiny root canals perfect for colonizing. With every bite down in the mouth the pressure pumps the spirochetes throughout the body from these nests.

Q. What about antibiotics?

A. According to the US Food and Drug Administration (FDA), ciprofloxacin, gemifloxacin, levofloxacin, moxifloxacin, norfloxacin, and ofloxacin are six antibiotics that can cause permanent nerve damage.

These antibiotics can cause damage to tendons and organs such as kidneys and eyes. One of the six antibiotics is subject to a number of complaints from patients who have suffered serious side effects.

Whether taken orally or by injection, the resulting permanent nerve damage, such as peripheral neuropathy and damage to hands and feet, can result in symptoms like pain, tingling, numbness, weakness, fever and decreased or increased sensitivity to the sense of touch. Therefore the use of these drugs should be carefully considered.

Q. How important is it to eat organic foods?

A. Leaky gut comes about after we ingest GMO- and pesticide-laden foods. These pesticides act to make the bugs stomach explode. When we ingest these same plants the pesticide is still contained within. It acts like a grenade in our intestines blowing holes into the semipermeable intestinal lining. Think of it as your porch screen. When the holes are the proper size the breeze flows in and out easily, while keeping bugs outside. When leaky gut hits the scene the screen is torn with large holes throughout. From there undigested food particles and fecal matter escape into the bloodstream causing dirty blood. These dirty particles lodge around the body and the yeast within them proliferate causing greater health concerns. Inflammation is a warning sign that something big needs to shift. This shift is a lifestyle process not an event. Wash all fruits and vegetables from the store and buy organic as much as possible to minimize exposure to this health concern. One note that if you buy your organic vegetables and fruits from a local farmers market it will have natural beneficial bacteria on it. Rinse produce to remove surface dirt but try to maintain the added garden soil goodies.

Q. Does Lyme make you sensitive to beef?

A. Yes. Even blood tests show it. They have shown those who have been bitten by ticks are allergic to beef due to a specific protein. Eating organic pumpkin seeds and walnuts, and drinking black cherry juice is very beneficial.

Forget pork all together. Pigs do not have sweat glands and eat garbage and poop. That all stays in their system and they have the deadliest tapeworm parasites!

Q. What if I am also diagnosed with other issues such as megaloblastic anemia, Hashimoto's disease, low iodine, low estrogen, low progesterone, low cortisol, or MTHFR 1298?

A. It is all about *hope* and *faith* and finding the sunny-side up! You have the knowledge and desire. MTHFR is very difficult. A good-quality glutathione deserves consideration. One word of caution regarding glutathione: if you are sensitive to sulfur, then glutathione should possibly be avoided. A comprehensive lifestyle and nutritional evaluation would be needed to design a comprehensive health plan addressing these other health issues.

Antibiotics are only a temporary solution for many. From there one needs to dive deep into the inner terrain of the body to see which filtering system is blocked. This is also where prior body insults, both physical and emotional, harbor acidic environments perfect for the Lyme breeding ground.

Q. I have had severe back and joint pain. I had hip surgery thinking it would help … it did not. Brain fog, poor concentration, headaches, forgetfulness, stuttering, fatigue and balance issues, and twitching. I had a bite on the back in 2007; the doctor said it looked like staph. Test came back negative, and no further tests were done. I've had issues since then, getting worse. I have been to so many doctors.

A. It is so difficult and painful. Those were many of my symptoms. By now you realize there are many false positive/negative tests. The tools listed here in this book will help calm the inflammation of the inner terrain. The next step is to stop ingesting toxins such as sugar, processed foods, smoking and stimulants like coffee. Dealing with brain fog and stuttering, we will want to reduce the heavy metal toxicity in the body incorporating leafy green foods. Boost best quality probiotic intake. Every day try to do something special toward cleaning up the diet. Eat organic as much as possible. We all say we cannot afford it, yet a side-by-side price comparison between a Snickers bar versus an avocado shows that each one on average is $1.49. It always comes down to our choices.

Sugar encourages colony growth, and the pain we feel is our body cleaning up the cellular debris after the colony die-off, otherwise known as Herxheimer reaction. Colon hydrotherapy is a great tool for maintaining a clear elimination channel.

Q. If a person has *Bartonella* bacteria, does that mean they have Lyme? Could a person have *Bartonella* but not have Lyme?

A. It has been my personal experience that these are two distinct diseases. *Bartonella bacilliformis* was the first species discovered. Then there are other *Bartonella* bacteria disease agents. All have been infecting humans for more than four thousand years. Often Bartonella is very debilitating and misdiagnosed, cat scratch fever is an infection which produces an ugly, bone-gnawing, searing, striking pain and can be even worse than Lyme. You can have one without the other. For reliable Bartonella testing contact Galaxy Testing; email: contact@ galaxydx.com.

Q. Why should I detox?

A. Your body has an amazing filtering system. Keeping our filtering organs clear allows our immune system to work efficiently. If we can manage to get out of our own way this will happen naturally through the body's own wisdom and knowing. For example if you are stopping a stimulant like sugar you might experience a radical difference in available energy. In the past your body used sugar for an energy boost which is usually followed by an energy let down. Without sugar your body will now rely on its own resources for energy and for a while you may feel more tired and less energetic. This tired feeling is the newly discovered natural balance of our own adrenal strength. We are so used to banging on our adrenals to push forward and overextending our organ function with toxic overload, that we do not recognize our true nature. As we clear out toxins from our system, our new quiet and calm vibrations strike us as curious and noteworthy and worth preserving. Our cells get addicted to cortisol baths invoked from constant trauma and drama in a chaotic lifestyle. Quiet rest is essential to reverse this stress.

Q. How can I prepare my yard for tick and flea prevention?

A. As for your immediate concern regarding our surrounding environment, cedar wood chips provide an excellent barrier border. Spreading diatomaceous earth around the yard, lawn, and garden will kill off ticks and fleas. Be sure to wear a mask as these pulverized shell particles can affect the lungs like asbestos. Once on the ground it is harmless. Check yourself and others every day for ticks. They can even be carried by the wind. Ask for peaceful cooperation with Mother Nature in completing the circle of life

Chickens will eat ticks in the yard if you feel so inclined. Fresh eggs would be wonderful. Today I have enough energy to care for chickens but while I was recovering that was not an option. If we approach Lyme as a virus, eggs are not advised as they feed viruses.

Q. How do you manage overwhelming fear and loss of faith in your life?

A. Living a balanced life shows up when we wake up first thing in the morning. If we are 100 percent restored, we wake up refreshed and light. But if we wake up thinking of drama and issues, then our energy reserves are scattered before we even get out of bed. Before getting out of bed each day take a moment to awaken slowly. Stretch, breathe deeply and exhale and focus your quiet mind on yourself for a spell. Then arise purposefully and move calmly into your day. Got kids jumping in bed with you? Teach them to meditate. Have to walk the dog? Step on the earth with barefoot and reset your negative ions.

Fear and faith are two different sides of the same coin. One cannot exist at the same time as the other. Fear not. Yet keep the faith that you will fully recover.

Q. What are your practices surrounding limiting EMF exposure?

A. Do not use a microwave or an electric blanket; turn off router when not in use; each evening turn off unused breakers; sleep in a peaceful environment without TV, phone, computer, or blue lights. Ground to outdoors with bare feet on earth or rock, being aware of potential tick exposure when necessary. Sleep on grounding sheets and unplug nightstand lights. Instead of holding a cell phone or wireless phone, use a speaker phone and earphones with long cables.

As you work toward the goal of reducing all EMF exposure you will have greater results on the healing journey. Regarding electric blankets, my strategy plan explains that spirochetes grow at night. You are providing an irresistible incubating space for the spirochetes. The best compromise is to heat the bed with the blanket before you get in. Have it plugged into a timer set to shut-off before you get in bed. Be sure to unplug the electric blanket when you are ready to get in bed if there is still electricity running past the timer.

Q. What is one of the most important things that improved for you?

A. Prayer and meditation were wonderful for energy healing and regeneration each morning. My healing journey was only possible through beholding the healing powers of our Lord. It helped my healing most by listening to those who share their gift of love through scripture. Paul Nison at rawlife.com helped me understand the health laws in the Bible. It was wonderful to experience the positive results after applying this ancient blessed knowledge. I also listened to Pastor Arnold Murray of Shepherds Chappel for true Bible translations.

We are experiencing a death and rebirth process with this healing journey requiring letting go of outmoded thoughts and behaviors which no longer serve us. By letting go we create a new space for allowing positive energies to enter and lift us up. As with anything, transformation through the death and rebirth process can be emotionally painful. Allow it to flow through you. Relaxing deeper to allow the new energy to flow in. Change is a process not and event.

Q. I feel like Lyme wins if I surrender. It feels like I am giving up.

A. There came a time when I understood that these little creatures were
   of God's Kingdom too. They were just surviving and living their
   Karma which plays a big role in life. It was not personal. I called on
   our Lord to help me move through this healing journey with as little
   damage as possible to myself and all beings.

This act of surrender is not about taking mental/emotional issues and
just switching to surrender. That makes no sense. It is not about giving
up and loosing, while we are letting the spirochetes win. It is more
that we surrender to the fact that all living beings are interdependent.
Each living being has a special role in life on this planet. The Lyme
spirochete's role is to help deer antlers grow. They are temporarily
misplaced in our bodies. Acceptance of this curable situation relieves
the need for blame. This too shall pass dear one.

Q. What is surrender to you?

A. Surrender is to a higher purpose by focusing on alignment, moment
   by moment. Follow the path of least resistance. Where there are
   blocks, gently realign and continue moving forward. Turning it over
   and over and over and yet again, turning it over each time with
   loving forgiveness as we grow in light.

Q. Is there an order of recovery from Lyme disease and co-infections
   with your protocol?

A. Yes there is an order. One must have patience.

   1) Lyme disease
   2) Fibromyalgia
   3) Chronic fatigue
   4) Rebuilding strength
   5) Reaching for the stars regaining empowered vitality

Over the recovery journey one stage blends gradually into another. The disease is on the run. One day at a time our ability to interpret our body's signals will grow and we can respond with self-care.

The beginning is slow. Keep at it in a determined and focused way. The pain-free times will start to last longer and longer. Of course there are periods of setbacks. Work the program, adding to it with steady continuity.

Next the healing will start to accelerate. Now it keeps getting better and better. I have fully recovered to a healthy state of vitality.

Q. What if someone does not have the will to survive and thrive?

A. I see this as a mind vs heart matter. The mind does get tired. It is fear based and anxiety ridden when under Lyme's tyranny. The Heart never tires and it never gives up. Look how beautifully it keeps time. Lyme can physically damage the heart and it can attack the mind and hold it hostage but it can never kill our Spirit. To calm the mind remove inflammatory toxins of all kinds. To heal the physical heart have proper nutrition, plenty of sunshine, fresh air and aerobic exercise under a doctors care. I recently participated in an 8 Weeks to Wellness program at my chiropractors office and I am so pleased with the complete overhaul of my system, head-to-toe. I gained back 1" in height, my emotional roller-coaster ride stopped, lingering digestive issues completely cleared. My confidence is back and I made wonderful new friends. That is a win-win in my book.

Q. Have you given yourself permission to heal?

A. This is a serious question which should be given serious thought. Sometimes people actually get a benefit from being sick. Perhaps they find the attention they crave with special care, or it keeps them from dealing with other unpleasant realities which they feel are out of their control. Sometimes they are done with their mission in this lifetime. Perhaps it is their time to drop the physical body and operate from non-physical reality. Only you will know your truth.

Find that truth and give yourself permission to follow your heart's desire.

Q. Are you willing to ignore all the naysayers and do whatever it takes to overcome this illness?

A. I know, right! At first I was super sensitive about the periodic haters who would come after my posts of healing on Facebook. Because some of the comments were so mean, I decided to open my own private FaceBook group call The Gift Of Lyme Disease and Co-Infections. You are all invited to send me a friend request at Suzen Chan and I will add you to this private page. I have a case that had to go through the court system so I have lots of doctors, lawyers, judges and the like to back up my level of disability and that I did recover after years of suffering. And believe me the insurance companies wanted me eviscerated and dead. As a veteran multiple modality healer, I was able to figure this out and heal myself. I know you can do this too!

REFERENCES

IGENIX, Inc.

www.Igenex.com

LYME Testing Western blot

795 San Antonio Rd
Palo Alto, CA 94303
800.832.3200
650.424.1191
650.424.1196 Fax

GALAXY DIAGNOSTICS, INC.

www.galaxydx.com

BARTONELLA Testing

For general inquiries:

Call: 919-313-9672
Fax: 919-287-2476
Email: contact@galaxydx.com
Hours: 9-5pm, Monday – Friday

Courier Address

Galaxy Diagnostics, Inc.
7020 Kit Creek Rd, Ste 130
Morrisville, NC 27560

USPS Mailing Address

Galaxy Diagnostics, Inc.
PO Box 14346
Research Triangle Park, NC 27709

ABOUT SUZEN

SUZEN IS A pioneering multiple modality therapeutic healing practitioner. Her unique and extensive research and techniques have allowed her to discover the profound interdependent integrative nature between body, mind and spirit. Suzen reveals the simple accessible tools needed to heal an ailing humanity. She has successfully healed conditions once thought incurable, irreversible, or unchangeable releasing individuals from life sentences of suffering. Through her studies in the United States, Czechoslovakia, China and Tibet, Suzen holds over thirty-three certifications in advanced healing in the fields of Licensed Massage Therapy; Colon-Hydro Therapy; Counseling Holistic Healing Practitioner, Detox and Regeneration Therapy Specialist.

Being a healing spiritual catalyst Suzen cured herself of Chronic Neurological Lyme Disease and Co-Infections after the doctors report claimed she would never work again. Suzen is now dedicated to bringing hope and help to those still suffering with this debilitating chronic disease. Lyme is the activator paving the way for a new healing paradigm. This new way of healing calls to those who believe the answer lies within their own power and are willing to do the work necessary for recovery.

Thank you for your purchase.

To register for your Free Gifts please read below:

YOUR FREE GIFTS

Thank you for purchasing <u>The Gift of Lyme Disease and Co-Infections;</u> <u>A Healer's Journey to Healing Lyme,</u>

To show my appreciation I would like to give you free gifts to help you get your Lyme Journey started right away!

To register for your free gifts please go to <u>www.TheGiftOfLymeDisease.com</u> where you can receive your free gifts and start feeling better now.

by grace,

Suzen